ALZHEIMER'S DISEASE DECODED

The History, Present, and Future of
Alzheimer's Disease and Dementia

ALZHEIMER'S DISEASE DECODED

The History, Present, and Future of Alzheimer's Disease and Dementia

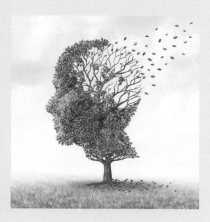

Ronald Sahyouni
UC Irvine

Aradhana Verma
UC San Francisco

Jefferson Chen
UC Irvine

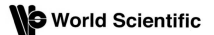
World Scientific

NEW JERSEY · LONDON · SINGAPORE · BEIJING · SHANGHAI · HONG KONG · TAIPEI · CHENNAI · TOKYO

Published by

World Scientific Publishing Co. Pte. Ltd.
5 Toh Tuck Link, Singapore 596224
USA office: 27 Warren Street, Suite 401-402, Hackensack, NJ 07601
UK office: 57 Shelton Street, Covent Garden, London WC2H 9HE

Library of Congress Cataloging-in-Publication Data
Names: Sahyouni, Ronald, author. | Verma, Aradhana, author. | Chen, Jefferson, author.
Title: Alzheimer's disease decoded : the history, present, and future of Alzheimer's disease and
    dementia / Ronald Sahyouni, Aradhana Verma, Jefferson Chen.
Description: New Jersey : World Scientific, 2016. | Includes bibliographical references and index.
Identifiers: LCCN 2016033859| ISBN 9789813109247 (hardcover : alk. paper) |
    ISBN 9813109246 (hardcover : alk. paper) | ISBN 9789813109254 (pbk. : alk. paper) |
    ISBN 9813109254 (pbk. : alk. paper)
Subjects: | MESH: Alzheimer Disease | Dementia
Classification: LCC RC523 | NLM WT 155 | DDC 616.8/31--dc23
LC record available at https://lccn.loc.gov/2016033859

British Library Cataloguing-in-Publication Data
A catalogue record for this book is available from the British Library.

Printed in Singapore by Mainland Press Pte Ltd.

Najib Okko,

And all those who lost their lives to Alzheimer's disease.

Contents

About the Authors   ix

Building a Community   xv

Foreword   xvii

Preface   xix

Quick Reference Guide   xxvii

Part I: Introduction, History, and Overview   **1**

Chapter 1:   Introduction to the Brain and Nervous System   3

Chapter 2:   Dysfunction   31

Chapter 3:   Senility and Normal Aging   49

Chapter 4:   What is Dementia?   59

Chapter 5:   Introduction to Alzheimer's Disease   73

Chapter 6:   Epidemiology of Alzheimer's Disease   99

Chapter 7:   The History of Alzheimer's Disease   121

Chapter 8:   An Interesting Link   139

Part II: Novel Therapies and Future Directions   **153**

Chapter 9:   Surgical Treatments for Dementia   155

Chapter 10:   Is There a Link to Traumatic Brain Injury?   165

Chapter 11:   What's going on Now?   175

Chapter 12:   Novel Therapies   191

Chapter 13:   How Can We Solve the Problem?   221

Chapter 14:   What Resources Exist?   235

Acknowledgements   245

Note to Readers   247

Glossary/Abbreviations   249

Index   255

About the Authors

Ronald Sahyouni

Biography

My interest in the brain developed early on, during a wonderful psychology class I took in high school. This interest became realized and personalized when I watched my grandfather die of Alzheimer's disease. This heartbreaking experience made me hope to never again see anyone die of such a disease, and although this hope may be unrealistic, it has led me to fight towards reaching a goal of a world without Alzheimer's disease. After high school, my undergraduate studies took place at the University of California, Berkeley, double majoring in Neurobiology and Psychology in order to understand the brain at a microscopic and systemic level. Concurrently, I worked at the University of California, Davis Alzheimer's Disease Center, conducting neuropsychological evaluations of patients who were referred to our research clinic. These experiences taught me that there was a tremendous lack of progress being made in treating Alzheimer's disease, which pushed me to pursue a career as a physician scientist. This brought me to the Medical Scientist Training Program (MSTP; an MD/PhD program) at the University of California, Irvine School of Medicine, where I have been fortunate to participate in a variety of projects aimed at better understanding the brain, from traumatic brain injuries (TBI) and brain tumors to Alzheimer's disease.

Why Alzheimer's disease?

I remember looking into my grandfather's eyes when I was an 8-year-old kid in elementary school and seeing the wisdom, understanding, experience and love that filled them. I remember the day that he was diagnosed with Alzheimer's disease, and I remember watching the brilliant light that echoed from his soul dissipate into absolute and irrevocable darkness. I saw his steadfast mind became unsure and wandering, with a steady decline in spatial memory and losing his way in familiar places. I wanted to pursue my intellectual curiosity and explore the world of Alzheimer's disease. Along my journey, I met an unfortunately sizeable population of individuals afflicted with a disease that truly tore apart the substance of sentience. I have also been fortunate to meet a correspondingly sizable and motivated populace of individuals who have dedicated their lives to ridding the world of Alzheimer's.

Aradhana Verma

Biography

I have a Masters in Translational Medicine (MTM)under the Bioengineering Department of UC Berkeley and UC San Francisco. As part of my Masters project, I chose to dedicate my time to the development of a wearable device to help patients with dementia. The device would have a monitoring system, communication tools and games to keep patients safe and engaged. It sounded like the perfect tool to help patients suffering from memory issues until there was a treatment for dementia and Alzheimer's disease. It was during this period that I began to interact with clinicians and patients in order to understand the reality of dementia. This reality startled me. Neurologists, gerontologists and caregivers seemed exhausted by the battle. Patients were often not motivated enough or sufficiently cognizant to face their disease. We concluded that this chronic condition was not amenable to a technological intervention, or at least not now. Up until then, my perception of modern medicine included prosthetics, regenerative medicine, and personalized devices. I saw medicine as an active form of care and treatment. This was my first reluctant experience of palliative care. As a team, we made a decision to change gears and consider an acute disease in which the science was better understood — stroke. While our assigned project changed, my interest in dementia and Alzheimer's disease only grew.

Why Alzheimer's disease?

During my undergraduate years at UC Berkeley, I had the opportunity to work with my supervisor-turned-mentor, Dr. Tandis Vazin, on modeling Alzheimer's disease and other neurodegenerative diseases using human embryonic stem cells. Concepts of "neurogenesis" and "cellular restoration" were constantly brought up in conversations, experimental designs, and publications. As an aspiring researcher, I was truly optimistic that the pathologies and traumas of Alzheimer's disease would soon be gone. I wanted to be at the frontier of the battle against this disease, a battle I was sure we would win during my lifetime.

Within Alzheimer's disease, I am learning about ongoing clinical trials, understanding the paradigm of care globally, and scrutinizing the progress that has been made. I am beginning to understand the need for palliative care, but I also believe that we are closer to a cure with every trial, every drug and each new advocate in the field. I hope to raise awareness and advocacy with each new reader of this book.

Dr. Jefferson Chen

Biography

I have been fascinated by the brain and its functions from my early neuroscience studies during my undergraduate training at the California Institute of Technology. The basic science studies there served me well as I continued my MD/PhD training at the Johns

Hopkins University School of Medicine, where my graduate studies were directed at the molecular and cellular biology of lysosomes and the endocytic pathways. This was an interesting time in the late 1980s, during which there was a flourishing of the neurosciences and an explosion in knowledge in molecular neurochemistry. I went on and did my neurosurgery residency at the University of California, San Diego, and had an outstanding exposure to studies directed at the basic molecular underpinnings of neurological disorders such as traumatic brain injury (TBI) and Alzheimer's. During the 5 years on the faculty at the University of Texas Medical Branch in Galveston and subsequent 15 years at the Legacy Emanuel Medical Center in Portland, Oregon, my focus in clinical and basic research has been directed at the surgical treatment of TBI acutely with novel surgeries and intense multimodal brain monitoring in the intensive care unit. During my time in Portland, I had the privilege of being the neurosurgeon for the pivotal multicenter Alzheimer's Cognishunt trial (Portland site). Involvement in this trial not only taught me about the intricacies of dementia, but also gave me a first-hand appreciation of the devastating toll of Alzheimer's on patients and their families.

Why Alzheimer's disease?

In my current role as the medical director of neurotrauma at the University of California, Irvine, I have continued my focus on the early treatment of patients with traumatic brain injury, with an emphasis on therapy guided by multimodal brain monitoring in addition to radiographic and clinical data, but there is much more to do. The prevalence of mild traumatic brain injury (TBI) and concussions is staggering, and their relationship with Alzheimer's is epidemiologically established, but the molecular mechanisms are still areas of intense study. I have also spearheaded a Normal Pressure Hydrocephalus (NPH) initiative and an initiative to develop new paradigms for the treatment of chronic subdural hematomas, both of which being neurosurgically treatable entities that mimic Alzheimer's. The recent findings regarding brain lymphatics also provide new avenues of clinical and basic study as to their role in cerebrospinal fluid (CSF) circulation, which may ultimately affect the β-amyloid depositions that are characteristic of Alzheimer's. We hope to be pioneers in these endeavors.

Building a Community

The fight against Alzheimer's disease is a fight that an entire community undertakes together. For patients and their families, it is a battle that necessitates the use of medical treatment as well as modifying lifestyles in order to minimize the risk of diagnosis and deterioration of the disease. This includes taking medications, getting enough sleep, relaxing in an attempt to decrease perceived stress, exercising and eating the right foods. Together, these actions synergistically fight the disease. For researchers, this means collaborating on results — both good and bad — and understanding the disease through many, many disciplines. Similarly, this disease requires that we build an interdisciplinary community and support one another. So in addition to delivering this book, we, the authors, would like to build upon the community that includes our readers, and so we have created a social media platform for you to receive groundbreaking information about new discoveries, studies, and interviews with leading scientists in the field.

Please follow us on:

- Facebook: www.facebook.com/AlzheimersDecoded
  - Link to YouTube through our Facebook page
- Twitter: www.twitter.com/AlzDecoded

Foreword

Dr. Federoff

Alzheimer's disease (AD) is the scourge of this century. AD has varied etiology, dichotomized by genetic contribution. Familial AD (FAD), caused by coding region mutations in three genes, is quite rare and characterized as a Mendelian form. The vastly more prevalent late onset AD (LOAD), is genetically complex and also implicates non-genetic factors as etiologic contributors.

While both FAD and LOAD share pathogenic, neuropathology, and clinical features it is clear that the different etiologic factors commend the scientific and clinical communities to consider them related but distinct entities. This recognition has profound implications for research, drug discovery and development and the emergence of future disease modifying therapeutics.

There are many active and important investigative issues currently facing the AD community. Among the most salient is to determine the range of etiologic factors that conspire with the inherited vulnerability component to produce manifestations of the disease. It is presumed that environmental factors are contributory; however, data linking antecedent exposures or experiences are still nascent. Perhaps the strongest case can be made for antecedent head injury. Mild to moderate traumatic brain injury (TBI) appears to underlie some later forms of cognitive impairment and dementia and neuropathologically define chronic traumatic encephalopathy (CTE). While both AD and CTE share beta-amyloid deposition and tauopathy, the anatomic distributions are distinct. Nonetheless, further characterization of mechanisms that link head trauma and later emergence of pathobiological features and clinical dementia warrant further study.

Additionally, the linkage between insulin resistance and type II diabetes mellitus (T2DM) with increased body mass index (BMI) suggest another environmental risk factor. Whether certain diets are independent contributors to AD risk or manifest the risk through systemic inflammation accompanying metabolic syndrome and T2DM are not yet clear. However, given the epidemic of obesity in the US and globally, this association portends possible increased rates of AD and perhaps presenting at a younger ages. This is a population health and policy issue with economic implications of unprecedented magnitude.

The large-scale failure of clinical trials, estimated at greater than 95%, in manifest AD and prodromal mild cognitive impairment (MCI) demand other approaches. One clear opportunity is to evaluate candidate investigational agents in the earliest stages of AD. Some clinical investigators believe that this should be done in the preclinical state. Efforts to define biomarkers of preclinical AD are essential in order to advance clinical trials in those at risk for AD.

This volume comprehensively reviews AD from many perspectives. The goals to fully describe the nature of AD, pathologies, current treatments, novel insights into pathogenesis and investigational approaches to modify natural history of AD are well met. This volume should appeal to anyone interested in Alzheimer's disease, regardless of background, from practitioners to the lay audience.

Howard J Federoff, MD, PhD
Vice Chancellor, Health Affairs
University of California, Irvine
CEO, UCI Health System

Preface

Alzheimer's disease has become a landmark disease of our aging global population, and an increasingly problematic public health menace. Unlike many other disorders, Alzheimer's disease largely affects not only the afflicted individual, but also puts significant emotional and financial burden on their friends, family, and the community. All approved treatments only marginally enhance cognitive performance in affected individuals. Hundreds of failed clinical trials reflect the enigmatic pathology that underlies Alzheimer's disease. We want to tell the story of the scientists, physicians, and patients who have been waging a war against Alzheimer's disease, and also pay homage to those who have lost their lives in the process.

This war has many fronts — from the personal and political efforts focused on ending Alzheimer's disease, to the scientific battles being fought in order to change the trajectory of cognitive deterioration in patients living with Alzheimer's. After we began working on this book, we worked hard to learn of the stories of the people around us and their personal experiences with Alzheimer's disease. Almost everyone we spoke with had a personal story related to Alzheimer's disease, whether it was their own parents, in-laws, or family friends who were affected. We were surprised to find that despite the prevalence and significance of Alzheimer's disease in our society, there was not a single book for the general public that succinctly covered the history, science, and future of the disease. Our hopes when writing this book were to convey the story of Alzheimer's disease, from its history to the reasons why efforts to treat the disease have been so difficult and unwieldy. It was our hope that any individual interested in Alzheimer's disease could use this book to better understand where we are scientifically, politically, and therapeutically in our fight to end Alzheimer's. The present stage in our battle is bittersweet; we do not yet have any Food and Drug Administration (FDA)-approved medications or therapies that are curative, yet there are many promising potential treatments on the horizon.

People who are familiar with our interest in Alzheimer's frequently ask us where we are in terms of successfully eradicating the disease. Doing a quick Google search or watching any health newsfeed will readily yield an abundance of news headlines and advertisements for the next "cure" to Alzheimer's disease. Many times, these claims are misleading or completely false — generally being predicated on homeopathic or unproven remedies. These claims of "cures" to an incurable disease are harmful to the scientific efforts to study the disease and its treatment. Oftentimes, these claims create a false sense of hope for the patients suffering from Alzheimer's disease and their families, while unfortunately being motivated by financial gain. By offering individuals living with Alzheimer's disease the promise of a cure, these pseudoscientists are failing the ethical and moral obligations of the scientific community to bring safe, proven, and evidence-based therapies to the market. We have received several phone calls from family members asking us what we think about the new cure discovered in country X, and after researching the claims made by the company producing the so-called "cure," we are constantly reminded of the duty of physicians and scientists around the world to "first do no harm" and not provide false hope to patients who are suffering from a terminal illness. But when it comes to the real science being done in laboratories around the world, the promise of a treatment is slowly being realized. Our belief that a treatment or cure for Alzheimer's disease will emerge is, in short, cautiously optimistic. Although at the present time there are no drugs, treatments, or voodoo techniques that can effectively ward off the progression of the disease, there are many promising therapies on the horizon. Currently, there are several FDA-approved drugs on the market that have been shown to improve cognitive performance in individuals with Alzheimer's disease; however, they fail to alter the pathological process underlying their cognitive deterioration. It is like using fire doors to stop a fire without actually addressing the underlying issue. However, the problem is that these drugs do not work as well as fire doors do.

Alzheimer's disease has proven itself to be a nearly insurmountable disorder, with hundreds of unsuccessful clinical trials worldwide.[1] Another major issue is that even if we were able to find a treatment, it is still extremely difficult for physicians to accurately predict which individuals will develop Alzheimer's disease and which will not. There is a lack of biomarkers that allow doctors to stratify patients based on risk, and since the earliest clinical symptoms do not bring the patient to the doctor's office until very late in the disease process, it is imperative that we are also able to diagnose Alzheimer's disease before it has taken its biological and cognitive toll on the brain. We cannot simply treat every patient once they turn 65, since any treatment yields a certain set of risks and side effects. We must be able to have some sort of understanding of the risk factors that certain individuals have and treat those with the highest risk prophylactically, while providing those who are at less risk with careful observation and yearly follow-ups. Fortunately, there is a lot of work being done on both sides of the coin, from early diagnosis using brain imaging, blood tests, and spinal taps, to groundbreaking therapies that use small molecules and stem cells in order to alter the course of the disease process.

In an ideal scenario, we would have comprehensive care clinics that would thoroughly screen individuals once they turned 50, just like the recommendation to receive a colonoscopy once you turn 50. Individuals who are at risk, whether based on family history, genetic risk factors, cardiovascular disease, or screening tests, could be candidates for further rigorous neuropsychological, genetic, and biological testing in order to better evaluate their risk for progressing to Alzheimer's disease. Those who are at risk would ideally be placed on prophylactic (preventative) medications that would slow the onset and progression of the disease, and individuals who are already expressing symptoms of cognitive decline would ideally be placed on disease-altering medications, once they are available. This is our vision for how Alzheimer's disease will be treated in the future, and it is one that many individuals in the field share. A comprehensive, personalized, and multi-disciplinary approach to the treatment of Alzheimer's is crucial to its successful eradication, and we truly believe that we will make significant progress towards this goal in the coming decades.

This book also seeks to explore the response of the United States and the global response to Alzheimer's disease. Globally, there are an estimated 46.8 million people living with dementia (a severe decline in mental function), with Alzheimer's disease being the cause of dementia in the majority of people. This enormous number is expected to double every 20 years, unless we find interventions. Much of the increase will happen in low- to middle-income countries.[2] Alzheimer's disease is thus a global crisis. We must all team up and rise above it.

It is well known that President Ronald Reagan was diagnosed and lived with Alzheimer's, but there are many more celebrities, world leaders, husbands, dads, moms, and loving family members who have lost their livelihoods due to this devastating illness.[3] The fight against Alzheimer's now has global backing, with the first-ever Global G8 Dementia Summit taking place in London. British Prime Minister David Cameron proclaimed that "we have stood against malaria, cancer, HIV, human immunodeficiency virus (HIV) and acquired immunodeficiency syndrome (AIDS) and AIDS — and we are just as resolute today. I want on December 11, 2013, to go down as the day that the global fight [against Alzheimer's disease and dementia] began."[4] The G8 Summit included representatives from the United States, UK, Canada, Germany, France, Italy, Russia, and Japan, with speakers ranging from Margaret Chan, MD (director of the World Health Organization) to Peter Dunlop, a patient and advocate with dementia.

Alzheimer's disease has evolved to become one of the most prevalent disorders afflicting seniors worldwide. In fact, nearly an entire branch of the US Government — the National Institute on Aging (NIA) — is focused on the study of Alzheimer's disease and dementia. Many countries have branches focused on dementia, such as the Medical Research Council of Great Britain and the European Union Joint Programme — Neurodegenerative Disease Research Initiative hosted by the European Commission. Yet despite the years of research, clinical trials, pharmaceutical advancements, and a cutting-edge understanding of brain function, Alzheimer's disease has managed to confound and evade every therapy that has sought to halt its progression. Fortunately, there are several excellent federal and non-profit resources that provide assistance to individuals suffering from Alzheimer's disease and their family members.

One of the premier non-profit agencies that seeks to bolster support and further the cause of Alzheimer's disease treatment is the Alzheimer's Association. On their website, there is a wealth of informational material, caregiver resources, and even links to clinical trial enrollment. If you or anyone you know is afflicted with Alzheimer's disease, we would encourage a thorough visit to the Alzheimer's Association website (www. alz.org). Another great resource for individuals looking to learn more about Alzheimer's disease or to help their family members or loved ones who are afflicted with the disease is the NIA's Alzheimer's Disease Education and Referral Center (www.nia.nih.gov/alzheimers). This website has a plethora of information related to Alzheimer's disease, and includes a toll-free number that can assist caregivers with any questions that they have or can provide help with navigating the website, as well as providing the opportunity to enroll in various clinical trials.

Another fantastic resource that we highly recommend to anyone dealing with Alzheimer's disease is a free informative book published by the NIA titled *Alzheimer's Disease: Unraveling the Mystery* — this 84-page manuscript provides an excellent overview of normal brain function, the abnormalities associated with Alzheimer's disease, updates on cutting-edge research, and caregiver resources. Being an informed patient, family member, or concerned citizen is crucial in the fight against

Alzheimer's. Since we are still in the earliest stages of truly understanding and curing Alzheimer's disease, a knowledgeable public and government can greatly impact the future of discoveries, therapeutics, and the course of Alzheimer's disease.

From an individual to a national level, understanding the impact that Alzheimer's disease has on the patient, their family, and the nation as a whole is crucial to the successful eradication of the disease. At the present stage, Alzheimer's disease is thought of as an incurable disorder due to its complexity, its ubiquitous pathology, and the pedigree of unsuccessful clinical trials that sought to eliminate the disease process; however, similar to other diseases that were once deemed incurable, as new scientific discoveries are made, we will be equipped with novel tools with which we can approach the treatment of the disease.

Alzheimer's disease has already claimed many lives, but there are many more that are at risk, and we as a nation cannot bear to watch the disease unfold from the sidelines. We must be active, by advocating, donating, researching, and continuing to provide care to the millions of individuals afflicted with this devastating disease. As we uncover the mysteries of the brain and unravel the perplexities of the pathological process underlying Alzheimer's disease, we will hopefully be able to rid the world of a disease that robs an individual of their most precious memories.

This book serves to convey the history of Alzheimer's disease, as well as being a comprehensive overview of the most promising therapies that may eventually be employed in the successful treatment of Alzheimer's. We also thought that it might be meaningful to share our own personal experiences with Alzheimer's disease, in order to shed light and pay homage to the day-to-day struggles that millions of individuals around the world face on a daily basis.

One thing to keep in mind as you read through this book, however, is that the war against Alzheimer's disease is constantly evolving. New discoveries are made on a regular basis, and the scientific knowledge we gather is dynamic. As such, there may be new discoveries, treatments, and therapies that may not be addressed by this book. Although great care was taken to cover the history, evolution of scientific understanding, and recent therapeutic advancements in the fight against Alzheimer's disease, please keep in mind that we are still in the early stages of our fight, and many things will change in the near future that will hopefully bring us one step closer to a cure.

Before we proceed, we want to leave you with a quote by surgeon and writer Atul Gawande, which hopefully embodies the spirit of our struggle with Alzheimer's disease. It is a fight that is worth fighting: "[A cure] is possible. It does not take genius. It takes diligence. It takes moral clarity. It takes ingenuity. And above all, it takes a willingness to try." We will find a cure, but in order to do so, we need to try, never quit, and always look forward while learning from the past.

References

1. Alzheimer's Association. (n.d.) Clinical trials for Alzheimer's disease and dementia. Alzheimer's Association Research Center. [http://www.alz.org/research/clinical_trials/find_clinical_trials_trialmatch.asp] [Accessed January 31, 2016].

2. Alzheimer's Disease International. (n.d.) World Alzheimer Report 2015: The global impact of dementia. [http://www.alz.co.uk/research/world-report-2015] [Accessed January 31, 2016].

3. Anderson J. (2015) 20 famous people with Alzheimer's. [http://www.aplaceformom.com/blog/10-celebrities-with-alzheimers-disease/] [Accessed January 31, 2016].

4. Stephens S. (n.d.) Neurology news: World leaders gather to fight Alzheimer's Disease. *Neurology Now*. [https://patients.aan.com/resources/neurologynow/index.cfm?event=home.showArticle&id=ovid.com%3A%2Fbib%2Fovftdb%2F01222928-201410030-00013] [Accessed January 31, 2016].

Quick Reference Guide

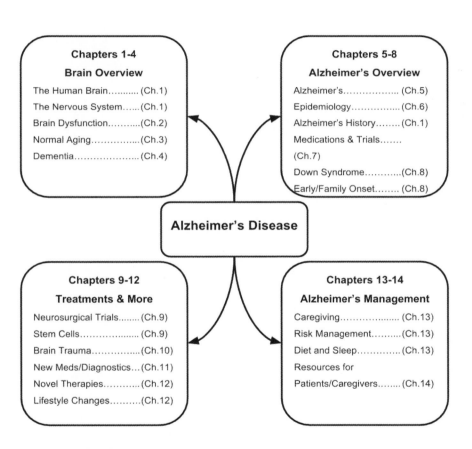

Chapters 1-4

Brain Overview

The Human Brain........... (Ch.1)

The Nervous System...... (Ch.1)

Brain Dysfunction.......... (Ch.2)

Normal Aging................ (Ch.3)

Dementia..................... (Ch.4)

Chapters 5-8

Alzheimer's Overview

Alzheimer's.................. (Ch.5)

Epidemiology................ (Ch.6)

Alzheimer's History........ (Ch.1)

Medications & Trials.......

(Ch.7)

Down Syndrome............ (Ch.8)

Early/Family Onset........ (Ch.8)

Alzheimer's Disease

Chapters 9-12

Treatments & More

Neurosurgical Trials........ (Ch.9)

Stem Cells.................... (Ch.9)

Brain Trauma................ (Ch.10)

New Meds/Diagnostics... (Ch.11)

Novel Therapies............ (Ch.12)

Lifestyle Changes.......... (Ch.12)

Chapters 13-14

Alzheimer's Management

Caregiving.................... (Ch.13)

Risk Management.......... (Ch.13)

Diet and Sleep.............. (Ch.13)

Resources for

Patients/Caregivers........ (Ch.14)

Additionally, please reference the glossary at the end of the book for a full list of abbreviations and definitions of commonly used terms.

Part I
Introduction, History, and Overview

1

Introduction to the Brain and Nervous System

"And this I believe: that the free, exploring mind of the individual human is the most valuable thing in the world. And this I would fight for: the freedom of the mind to take any direction it wishes, undirected. And this I must fight against: any idea, religion, or government which limits or destroys the individual."

— *East of Eden* by John Steinbeck, Nobel Laureate
(Literature, 1962)

The human brain is the most impressive structure Mother Nature has created. In fact, it is the most complex structure in the observable universe. It is capable of producing emotion, malleable enough to dynamically modify itself, and more powerful than any computer ever created. Despite these amazing feats, it consumes only 20 watts of energy (similar to a light bulb), is extraordinarily compact, and has mystified the greatest scientists in the history of humanity.

Life is interesting in that we are constantly exposed to dynamic sensory experiences — yet we rarely are aware of it. The brain is an organ that is able to recognize its own existence, which in itself is incredible. The fact that we are able to be consciously aware of ourselves, interact with other human beings in an incredibly complicated social landscape, produce machines and devices that are capable of artificial intelligence, and explore other planets is but a small homage to the brain's incredible capacity.

The brain is the seat of emotion and personality. It bestows us with individuality, our ability to empathize, contemplate the future, and recollect the past. When it is properly functioning, it truly is a miraculous system that is more capable than the world's largest and most powerful supercomputers.

The beauty of nature and the complexity of the world can be appreciated and comprehended by the brain. The sights and sounds of a bustling city are perceived by the very organ that created them, and we were somehow able to figure out how to leave the very planet from which the human brain evolved in order to explore our role in the universe. Beethoven's Fifth Symphony and the Mona Lisa were beautiful masterpieces of the brain. The human brain is continuously integrating and synthesizing data from the external environment, and producing a continuously seamless experience of consciousness. This results in a beautiful symphony of emotions, ideas, experiences, and beliefs that diversify and color the world around us. These feats are extraordinary to say the least, and they were all accomplished by an incredible population of humans thanks to the mass of cells within their skulls.

The human brain has the consistency of soft tofu, and despite the brain being so prolific, everything could be lost in the blink of an eye. During one of our many experiences working in the Neurosurgery Department at the University of California Irvine Medical Center, the team we were working with was called in to evaluate a trauma case that had just rolled into the emergency department (ED). The individual whom we saw was breathing lightly, was still wearing his regular clothes, and looked otherwise normal. The only abnormal thing about him was the fact that there was a massive hole in his skull from a self-inflicted gunshot wound. On the side where the bullet exited the skull was a hole with grayish material protruding from it — this was fresh brain matter that had left his skull due to the momentum of the bullet and the subsequent swelling within the cranial cavity. We threw some gloves on and one of the emergency room doctors asked us to try and clean up the brain matter and debris that was protruding from the bullet wound. As we did so, we were thinking just how soft and delicate the brain really is — and were reminded of just how incredible it is. Yet unfortunately, many people take its miraculous capabilities for granted. The patient that we were working on was eventually placed on artificial respiration since he was an organ donor, and after his organs were harvested the following day, he unfortunately died. He was in a vegetative state due to the massive amount of damage to his brain, and despite the fact that he had a perfectly functioning body, his mind was destroyed by the bullet's path, and the very organ that makes a human being was destroyed. Although in Alzheimer's disease the brain is not destroyed in the blink of an eye, the process is equally disruptive. The brain is what makes us who we are. As we continue to explore the brain, we are better able to understand how it works, and how it malfunctions in the case of Alzheimer's disease. However, prior to discussing Alzheimer's disease in detail, we will start with an overview of the human brain and the components that make it up.

Human Brain: Structure

The average human brain is 3 pounds (1,300–1,400 grams, about the weight of a bag of sugar or flour), or 2% of total body weight (Fig. 1.1). One study found that with increasing age, brain weight decreases by 2.7 grams in males and 2.2 grams in females per year.[1] Despite the brain making up such a small fraction of the total body weight, it is tremendously thirsty for nutrients, and 15% of the blood pumped by the heart (total cardiac output) goes to the brain. Additionally, the brain consumes 20% of the body's oxygen and 15% of total body glucose (sugar) due to its high metabolic demand.[2] The average human brain contains 100,000,000,000 (100 billion) brain cells (neurons), which is equivalent to the annual economic impact in dollars of Alzheimer's disease in the United States. Additionally, for each neuron, there are approximately 10 supporting cells (glial cells) — meaning that the average human brain has 1,000,000,000,000 (1 trillion) cells. What is even more astounding is the fact that each neuron makes hundreds and sometimes thousands of connections to other neurons in the brain, resulting in an incredible amount of complexity and refinement that is unparalleled by anything else in the universe.

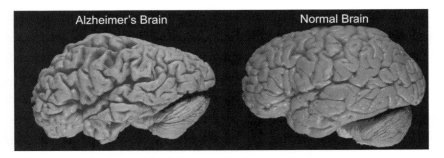

Fig. 1.1.   A normal brain (right) compared to a brain with Alzheimer's disease (left).[3] Note the drastic changes in size and shrinkage due to loss of brain cells in the Alzheimer's brain.

In order to function optimally, the brain has a built-in "filtration" system that removes toxic waste products and nourishes the brain. Cerebrospinal fluid (CSF) is a clear fluid found in the central nervous system (CNS), which includes the brain and spinal cord. The CSF is produced from the frond-like choroid plexus that resides within the cavities of the brain (Fig. 1.2). These cavities are called ventricles. CSF is also produced by the cells that make up the linings of the ventricles (known as the ependymal cells). After CSF is produced, it flows downwards through the brain from the lateral ventricles where it is formed, then to the third ventricle and through the aqueduct of Sylvius, and finally through the fourth ventricle at the bottom of the brain. As the CSF flows, it moves through what is known as the "subarachnoid space." This is a space that is found immediately above the brain and spinal cord, and is called "subarachnoid" because it is a space beneath — or "sub" — a protective layer of the brain known as the arachnoid. From the fourth ventricle, the CSF covers and nourishes the spinal cord, then flows over the surface of the brain, where it is reabsorbed back into the bloodstream. The reabsorption occurs thanks to what are known as "arachnoid granulations." These granulations protrude from the arachnoid that covers the brain and help reabsorb CSF that has already flowed through the CNS. While the primary function of CSF is to cushion the brain within the skull and

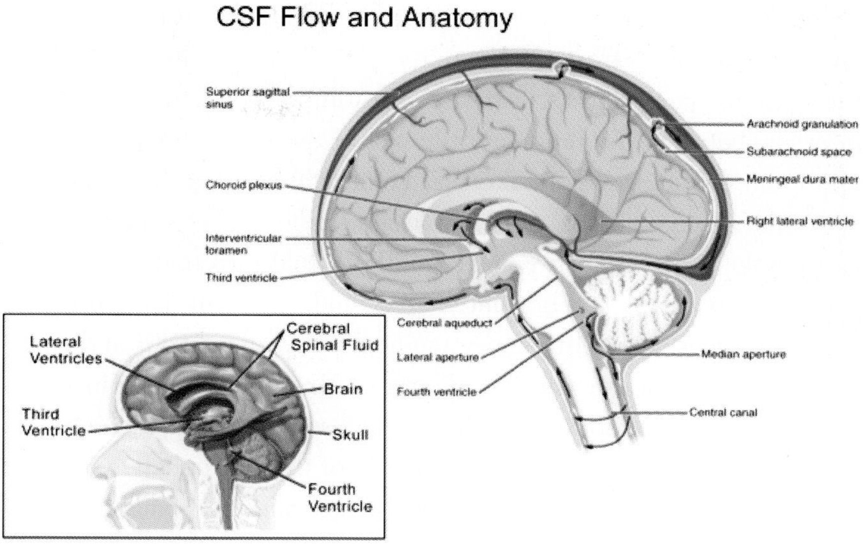

CSF Flow and Anatomy

Superior sagittal sinus
Choroid plexus
Interventricular foramen
Third ventricle
Arachnoid granulation
Subarachnoid space
Meningeal dura mater
Right lateral ventricle

Lateral Ventricles
Third Ventricle
Cerebral Spinal Fluid
Brain
Skull
Fourth Ventricle
Cerebral aqueduct
Lateral aperture
Fourth ventricle
Median aperture
Central canal

Fig. 1.2. Cerebrospinal fluid, or CSF, is produced by the choroid plexus and ependymal cells of the lateral ventricles → third ventricle → fourth ventricle → subarachnoid space over the brain and spinal cord → arachnoid granulations → reabsorption in venous blood. (Modified from Refs. 5 and 6.)

function as a shock absorber for the CNS, CSF also circulates essential nutrients that are filtered from the bloodstream and aids in the removal of toxins from the brain.

CSF is produced at a constant rate of 0.3 mL/min. This rate is equivalent to one drop of water dripping from an empty faucet every 3 seconds.[4] Interestingly, this rate of CSF production actually decreases in patients with Alzheimer's disease. Although the cause of this decrease is not entirely known, it may play a contributory role in the damaging effects of the disease. As CSF is produced, circulated, and reabsorbed within the brain, it helps nourish the cells within the brain, clear and filter out toxins (including the abnormal proteins found in Alzheimer's disease), and maintain the optimal environment for the proper functioning of brain cells.

During this cycle, CSF removes toxins from the brain. It does so by the one-way flow of CSF towards the bloodstream, where it is eventually reabsorbed and removed from the brain. In addition to removing toxins and waste products from the brain, the CSF transports hormones from the body to specific parts of the brain. Additionally, CSF provides an interface between the brain and the rest of the body, and serves as an important regulator of normality and homeostasis within the brain.

Since the year 2000, many published studies have found an important physiological link between CSF and the fluid surrounding the brain cells, known as the cerebral interstitial fluid. This link has prompted increased focus on a better understanding of the role of CSF in the normal brain, and more specifically, a better understanding of CSF in abnormal disease states. Additionally, the recent discovery of lymphatic vessels in the cranial cavity and the potential role of these lymphatic vessels in CSF absorption is changing our fundamental understanding of human neuroanatomy and brain function. Data have emerged that suggest that the newly discovered lymphatic vessels may play a role in CSF absorption. In fact, studies have sought to determine exactly where this interface between CSF and the lymphatic vessels may occur. The findings point to the cribriform plate and the nasal submucosa (structures found between the brain and the nose) as locations where CSF may be absorbed by lymphatics, thus transporting CSF to the venous system.[7] Interestingly, the bulk flow of CSF through the brain is aberrant in several neurological pathologies, including Alzheimer's disease and normal pressure hydrocephalus, and can lead to the abnormal accumulation of proteins.

In addition to the protective effects of CSF, the brain is covered by three layers of protective membranes known as meninges (specifically, the pia, arachnoid, and dura) (Fig. 1.3). The thickest and strongest meningeal layer is known as the dura mater. This term originates from the Medieval Latin root *"dura,"* which means tough, and *"mater,"* which means mother. The meninges help protect the brain, and when they are filled with CSF, they allow the brain to practically float in the CSF. A craniotomy is a neurosurgical procedure wherein a piece of the skull is removed to expose the underlying brain. The dura mater is immediately beneath the bone. Once this is incised and reflected, there are several layers of translucent meninges known as the arachnoid (discussed briefly earlier) and pia mater that cover the brain, but at this point, the surface of the brain can be visualized. This outermost surface of the brain is known as the cerebral cortex, and is what you probably visualize when you think of the brain. It resembles a walnut to a certain degree, due to its infoldings known as sulci and gyri. The reason that the brain, specifically the cerebral cortex, has so many grooves is to increase the surface area of the brain and thus increase the amount of cells that it can hold. Imagine taking a piece of paper and trying to fit it within a marble — in order to do so, the piece of paper would have to be crumpled up and would thus have lots of folds in order to fit it into such a small space. This increase in surface area allows the brain to contain many more cells than if it was a flat, unfolded surface.

The Nervous System

The nervous system is an extremely complex and critical system in the body. It is referred to as the "master control system" of the body and is related to nearly every component of physical and mental well-being. So what exactly is the nervous system?

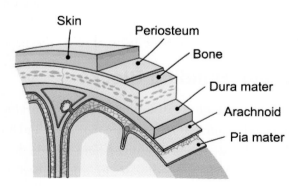

Fig. 1.3. The meninges are composed of the pia mater, arachnoid, and dura mater. They cover and protect the brain. Cerebrospinal fluid (CSF) flows in the "space" below the arachnoid, known as the subarachnoid space. (Figure credit: Ref. 8.)

An animal's nervous system consists of an intricate orchestration of individual nerve cells that coordinate all actions of the animal through complex biochemical and electrical signals. This highly integrated system consists of two major types of nerve cells, both of which are crucial to an animal's survival. The first and most well-known type of nerve cells are the neurons, which are directly responsible for the transmission of electrical and biochemical signals throughout the body. All of our thoughts, emotions, and behaviors can be broken down into three steps: sensation, integration, and action or reaction carried out by neurons.[9]

The second type of nerve cells are glial cells, which are actually 10-times more abundant than neurons. Glial cells can be subdivided into a few versatile categories, hosting crucial functions such as physical and structural support for the nervous system, maintenance, and regulation of the internal environment of the brain, protection of the neurons, and facilitation of neuronal action.

All of our neurons and glial cells are organized in two distinct, yet cooperative parts. The CNS (see Fig. 1.4), which consists of our brain and spinal cord, is the main control center of the body, while the peripheral nervous system (PNS; see Fig. 1.4), which consists of all of the nerves extending out from the brain and the spine, allows back-and-forth communication between the main control center and the rest of the body. We will explore the building blocks of the nervous system in the following section.

Human Brain: Building Blocks

The brain is able to accomplish extraordinary feats by working seamlessly in an interconnected manner. It is important to understand how the brain works normally, so that we can better understand how the brain malfunctions, as in the case of Alzheimer's disease. In order to better understand the entire brain, let us further explore all of the parts that make it up.

The smallest functional unit within the brain is on the order of a single cell. As previously described, cells within the brain are known as

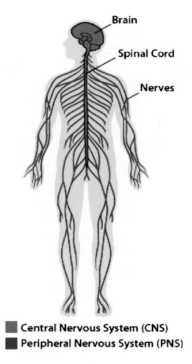

Brain

Spinal Cord

Nerves

■ Central Nervous System (CNS)
■ Peripheral Nervous System (PNS)

Fig. 1.4.   The central nervous system (CNS), shown in pink, consists of the brain and the spinal cord. The peripheral nervous system (PNS), shown in blue, consists of all of the nerves connecting the brain and spinal cord to all of the organs and muscles of the body. This image is not an exact representation of the brain or the nervous system. (Figure credit: Ref. 10.)

neurons, and these are the basic building block of the wide array of circuits that allow the brain to function. A cell is the basic building block of any organ in the human body. There are approximately 200 different types of cell in the human body, each of which is specifically optimized for a particular function depending on the body's needs. For example, a kidney cell is specifically designed to help filter fluid and extract useful nutrients and electrolytes that the body needs, while a heart cell specifically functions to contract in order to propel blood throughout the body.[11]

Each cell has unique properties and "substructures" known as organelles, which help facilitate the function of that individual cell.

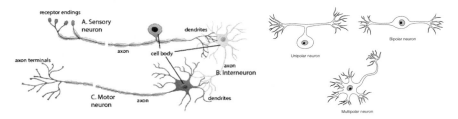

Fig. 1.5. Neurons typically consist of dendrites, a cell body, an axon, and axon terminals. In the right-hand image, we can see the three main types of neurons: unipolar, bipolar, and multipolar. In the left-hand image, we can see a unipolar sensory neuron (blue), sending information to a multipolar interneuron (yellow), which relays the information to the multipolar motor neuron (red). The specific neuronal connection shown in the left-hand image does not necessarily indicate a brain connection, thus it could be showing a simple involuntary response to stimuli such as the knee-jerk response: a tap to the knee is sensed by a sensory neuron on the muscle and relayed via an interneuron to a motor neuron to relax the muscle and allow the leg to extend. (Figure credit: Refs. 14 and 15.)

With regards to the brain, there are two primary cellular classifications: neurons and glia. A neuron (see Fig. 1.5) varies in size from 4 to 100 microns (0.004–0.1 mm) in diameter (a human hair is approximately 20 microns in diameter) and can transmit signals at speeds of 200 miles per hour.[12,13] Surprisingly, neurons can range in length from millimeters to over a meter (neurons that leave the spinal cord and innervate the lower extremities). Neurons are composed of a cell body known as a soma, which contains the important cellular organelles such as the nucleus, ribosomes, and rough endoplasmic reticulum (which functions in protein production), and more. The nucleus houses the cell's genetic information, and genes encode what is known as *messenger RNA (mRNA)*, which is then converted into proteins. Proteins are very important and serve many roles in the cell and body.

Neurons come in three main shapes and many different sizes. Specifics aside, their overall function is to sense the world around us, integrate and process the information we sense, and relay messages to our muscles and organs in order for us to react to our sensations. The neuron is able to receive signals from other neurons primarily through cellular extensions known as dendrites, and can transmit signals through a specialized extension known as an axon. The "end" of an axon is known as a synaptic bouton and usually forms a connection, or synapse, with the dendrite of another neuron. The synapse is where specialized chemicals, known as neurotransmitters, are released. These neurotransmitters can cause a variety of changes in the receiving neuron, and complex variations of neurotransmitter release help to create our experience of the world around us.

Bundles of axons in the periphery (outside the CNS) are known as nerves, or are known as tracts when they are within the CNS. Although neurons are the basis of neural circuits, the supporting cells play an equally important role in normal brain functions. These support cells, known as glial cells (derived from the word "glue"), were once thought to play only a small role in the brain. However, as more information was discovered about them, scientists began to recognize just how important they really are. Glial cells are critical in the formation of something known as the *blood–brain barrier*, which protects the brain from toxins. Glia also help with the removal of damaging substances from the brain and ensure a healthy extracellular environment for the neurons within the brain. Glial cells also function to promote the formation of new connections within the brain, and even help the brain to regenerate itself. They have even been implicated in the inflammatory response within the brain to various disease states, and in modulating the brain's ability to recover from trauma, strokes, infections, and much more.

Glial cells do not conduct neural impulses, but rather function to nourish and protect the neurons. Glial cells outnumber neurons 10 to 1 and are capable of regenerating, while neurons are generally unable to divide and renew. Glial cells are generally smaller than neurons and come in a variety of types (see Fig. 1.6), each of which is specialized for a particular set of functions. You may have heard the saying that we only use 10% of our brain. This inaccurate statement originated from the realization that glial cells outnumber neurons 10 to 1, and thus only

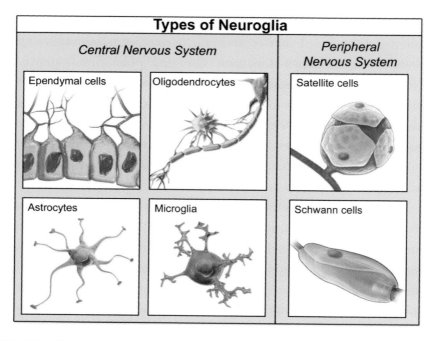

Fig. 1.6. There are various types of glial cells, also known as neuroglia, which support the nervous system. Ependymal cells line the ventricles within the brain and produce cerebrospinal fluid (CSF). Astrocytes help form the blood–brain barrier (BBB) and provide structural support for neurons. Microglia remove toxins and fight foreign invaders and are involved in inflammation and infection. Oligodendrocytes myelinate and insulate axons in the central nervous system (CCNS), while Schwann cells myelinate and insulate axons in the peripheral nervous system (PNS). (Figure credit: Ref. 16.)

10% of your brain is really made up of neurons, which are classically considered to be the quintessential "brain cell." In fact, we use 100% of our brain all the time. The entire brain is always metabolically active, and at times, we use certain parts of our brain or certain circuits more so than others and thus increase the metabolic activity of specific parts of the brain. However, at all times, even when you are sleeping or watching television, the entire brain is metabolically active and is working to synthesize and integrate new sensory stimuli with pre-existing knowledge and to maintain homeostasis throughout the body.

Neurons are specially equipped with the ability to form connections with one another. These connections, also known as synapses, are the molecular underpinnings of learning, language, emotion, and everything else that the brain produces (Fig. 1.7). These connections are constantly being made, modified, and destroyed. In fact, whenever you learn a new fact or concept, there are millions of new connections being formed, and your brain is literally being reorganized on a daily basis. These changes are microscopic in nature, but produce very visible macroscopic results. The brain's ability to dynamically modify itself confers upon it the ability to adapt to the environment and is also protective. This dynamic modifiability of the brain's neuronal networks and microscopic connections is known as "neuronal plasticity," and is one of the brain's most impressive attributes.

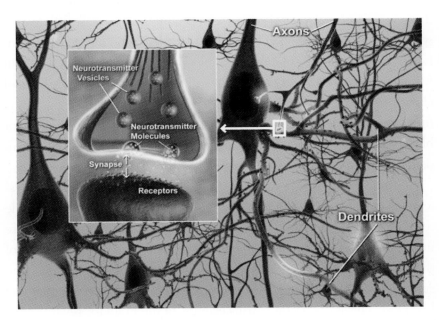

Fig. 1.7.   A graphic representation of neurons, their dendrites, and their axons, as well as the synapse (where the neurons communicate with one another via the release of neurotransmitters). (Figure credit: Ref. 17.)

Human Brain: Plasticity

The term "plasticity" is meant to connote pliability and malleability, analogous to a moldable piece of plastic. This implies that the brain can dynamically modify itself — changing the connections between circuits within the brain and synthesizing new connections on a daily basis. This provides the brain with a degree of resilience that allows it to protect and adapt itself to the environment. Plasticity is a normal part of the brain's day-to-day functioning, but it also comes in handy whenever the brain is damaged and needs to repair itself.

One common example in which neuronal plasticity is readily observed is in the case of stroke patients. A stroke is the neural equivalent of a heart attack. Usually, a blood clot or blockage occurs in one of the arteries that supplies blood to the brain. When blood flow is blocked, the part of the brain that artery supplies blood to is deprived of oxygen and nutrients, and there is an accumulation of toxic waste products. This causes the corresponding part of the brain to begin dying. If there is no medical intervention or spontaneous dissolution of the blockage, then that part of the brain will permanently die, and the patient will be left with varying degrees of clinical impairment. The impairment depends on the part of the brain, the size of the artery and the presence of collateral circulation to allow for blood circulation compensation. *Collaterals* are extra pathways or redundant blood vessels that are useful when the primary vessel is blocked.

Immediately after a stroke, patients usually exhibit profound physical or neurological alterations. For example, some patients are unable to move their arms or legs after an insult to the brain, while others are unable to speak. Neuronal plasticity is observed soon after the onset of the destructive processes of the stroke, however. Usually, patients who suffer a stroke are able to regain some degree of functionality that had been lost. This is due to the intrinsic ability of the brain to "rewire" itself and recognize what has been damaged. In addition to plasticity, there are some that argue that the improvement in function is the result of a decrease in local cerebral edema, which is swelling of the brain tissue.

Plasticity is an incredible characteristic that is unique to the brain and a few other organs (including the liver) within the body. Plasticity confers the brain with the ability to recover from injuries and learn new facts and skills, and is crucial for normal cognitive development. In fact, there are several cases of children who were born missing half of their brain and, to the amazement of physicians, were able to develop normally and have no apparent deficits.[18]

The cause underlying the ability of the brain to reprogram itself is that neurons are preprogrammed to fulfill a specific duty; however, they are able to modify their roles depending on the body's needs. In the case of individuals with massive neurological abnormalities, the brain is able to respond to the sensory input it is receiving and react in an appropriate manner. When an individual encounters the damaging effects of a stroke or has an entire half of the brain missing, the remaining neurons can decipher what roles they must fulfill in order to bring the body back to normal.

The degree of plasticity varies. It is most pronounced in children, but unfortunately diminishes with age. The reasons as to why neural plasticity is attenuated with age is multifaceted. It mainly has to do with a diminished number and robustness of neural stem cells that facilitate the regeneration of normal cognitive functions. This is why neurological insults later on in life can result in much more debilitation than a similar insult early on in the developmental process. Alternatively, some also argue that the older patient has had some loss of brain tissue over time and thus has less "reserve" for recovery. We will address this idea of cognitive "reserve" in the next chapter. A comparison of a brain scan of a young versus an older patient demonstrates an overall decrease in the volume of brain tissue in the latter (Fig. 1.8). There are also fewer stem cells available with age and thus the potential for plasticity is decreased.

Human Brain: Development

Recently, in order to understand how the brain functions in adults and elderly individuals, scientists have turned to early childhood

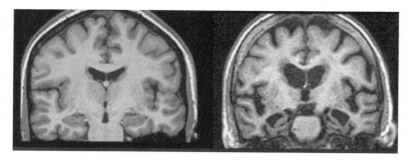

Fig. 1.8.   On the left is a magnetic resonance image (MRI) scan of a normal brain compared to a brain with Alzheimer's disease on the right. (Figure credit: Ref. 19.)

development in order to uncover the secrets of the origins of neural networks and consciousness. Consider how a newborn child is able to develop a literary library of several thousand words by the age of 4, around the same age that they begin to develop self-awareness and sentience.[20,21]

A newborn child's exploratory gaze invites billions of electrical impulses to synergistically tango in a dance that baffles scientists and is easily overlooked by many. A child's brain is exceptionally resilient, but also very sensitive to toxic substances such as alcohol or drugs. Upon birth, a child has an abundance of neurons that are primed for connectivity. As the child experiences life events, neural circuits begin to develop. However, excess neurons that are not activated or utilized will be destroyed upon birth, and are continuously destroyed until sexual maturation. This process is known as "synaptic pruning," and is thought to improve the efficiency of the human brain, removing unnecessary neurons and reinforcing important circuits.

Although there is a decrease in the number of neurons within the brain beginning at birth, the actual size of the brain increases by adulthood (Fig. 1.9). This increase in size is mediated by an increase in synaptic connectivity between neurons, as well as the myelination of neurons.[22] Myelin is a fatty "sheath" that covers axons and increases their ability to conduct neural impulses. This myelination begins in

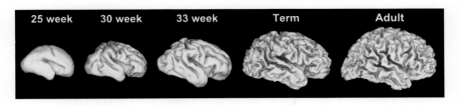

Fig. 1.9.   As the human brain develops, it becomes increasingly "folded" in order to maximize the surface area within the skull cavity. (Figure credit: Ref. 24.)

the 14th week of fetal development and continues until approximately 25 years of age.[23]

Synaptic pruning is affected by a variety of factors, primarily environmental, and can influence the synaptic density and number of neurons in the adult brain. Education, a stimulating environment, social interaction, and other early childhood exposures can influence the degree of synaptic pruning and ultimately the density of synaptic connections in the adult brain. A brain with dense connectivity has been suggested to be more resilient to diseases such as Alzheimer's disease, which destroys connections within the brain.[25]

Human Brain: Organization

The human brain, just like any architectural masterpiece, must have a blueprint. In general, the brain is divided into four lobes — the frontal, temporal, parietal, and occipital lobes — each of which is associated with distinctive functions (Fig. 1.10). For example, the occipital lobe, which is located in the hindmost part of the brain, is largely responsible for our sense of sight. The temporal lobes, which flank the sides of the brain, are generally responsible for our sense of hearing and ability to speak. However, the various lobes of the brain do not work in isolation. Rather, they are tightly interrelated, and are constantly communicating with one another and forming associations between the various lobes. These tight connections allow us to remember specific things in a multimodal way. For example, the first time you ever experienced pumpkin pie, you might have smelled the pie baking, heard the words "pumpkin pie," tasted the pie, and seen what the pie looked like. All of these disparate sensory stimuli somehow coalesced within the brain to create a single coherent concept of what pumpkin pie is. Now, when you think about pumpkin pie, you do not remember each individual sense in isolation, but rather you imagine a concept of the various aspects of pumpkin pie all integrated together to create a single cohesive experience. The brain does this thanks to the constant integration of sensations with pre-existing memories and experiences.

Apart from the four classic lobes, the brain has many more functional components. One of the key modules within the brain is an operational network known as the basal ganglia. This is a key regulator of emotion, personality, and memory. One important component of the basal ganglia is the hippocampus. The hippocampus can be thought of as the Holy Grail of memory. It is the site where new memories are formed. The role of the hippocampus was serendipitously discovered, and it turns out to be a major player in the early symptoms of Alzheimer's disease.

In a landmark clinical case, a patient known simply as H.M. (Henry Molaison) had his hippocampus surgically removed. The reason for the surgery was an attempt to treat H.M.'s intractable epilepsy. The foci of the epileptic seizures were thought to originate in the hippocampus. Thus, surgeons thought that by removing the hippocampus and surrounding structures, H.M.'s epilepsy would also be cured — and they were right. However, one major side effect became readily apparent — H.M. was no longer able to form new memories. He was no longer able to recognize new people that he had just met moments before, and he was unable to learn new facts.

Interestingly, other forms of memory remained functional — for example, motor learning, involving the ability to trace a figure using a pencil, was intact. H.M. was also able to recall memories and events that had taken place before his surgery. This unfortunate case allowed his physicians to deduce the role that the hippocampus played in learning

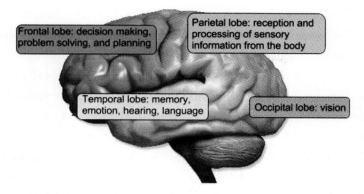

Fig. 1.10. The major lobes of the brain are highlighted — each serves a distinct set of functions. (Figure credit: Ref. 26.)

and memory. Interestingly, this is also the area that Alzheimer's disease is thought to attack first.

Human Brain: Memory and Integration

Neuroscientists have classified different types of memory into four categories: short-term, episodic, semantic, and procedural. Short-term memory is the ability to hold information in your mind that is immediately accessible for short periods of time. An example of this would be remembering a phone number that someone just gave you. Interestingly, this is usually the type of memory that is most affected by Alzheimer's disease early on. Episodic memory is the ability to store and recall autobiographical events, such as details regarding where you live and what your home looks like. This is the next type of memory that is adversely affected by Alzheimer's disease. Alzheimer's then attacks semantic memory, which is the ability to recall definitions and facts, such as the date of your family member's birthday or the definition of a word. Finally, procedural memory is the ability to perform tasks such as riding a bike or driving a car. This is the last type of memory to be destroyed by Alzheimer's disease. As memory becomes disrupted, other cognitive abilities such as spatial awareness, reasoning, language, attention, and problem-solving deteriorate.[27] As a patient develops Alzheimer's disease, they begin having difficulties in identifying or distinguishing between categories of objects, such as types of fruits or vegetables. Eventually, the inability to distinguish different types of fruits may extend to an inability to identify a fruit specifically, instead simply saying that it is a food item.

The hippocampus is an integral component of the formation of new memories (Fig. 1.11). The name hippocampus is derived from Greek and Latin roots meaning "seahorse," which, surprisingly enough, is what the hippocampus looks like in cross-section. This small functional component of the brain is crucial to the creation and synthesis of new memories with pre-existing knowledge. When it is lesioned or destroyed, patients are unable to form new memories, as in the case of patient H.M. Interestingly, old memories are spared. The reason for this is that older memories are actually ubiquitously stored throughout the cerebral cortex, which is the surface of the brain. The formation of new memories relies on the hippocampus, but once the memory is stored, the role of

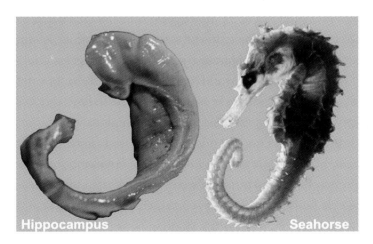

Fig. 1.11. The hippocampus (left) is derived from Greek and Latin roots meaning "seahorse" (right). (Figure credit: Ref. 28.)

the hippocampus becomes negligible. This is seen clinically in Alzheimer's disease, in which the hippocampus is one of the first regions of the brain to be affected by the disease process. As such, the hallmark clinical finding in Alzheimer's disease is memory difficulties — not problems recalling old childhood memories and important life events (at least not in the early stages), but rather problems with learning and the formation of new memories. Exactly how memories are made, stored, and integrated with prior knowledge is elusive; however, there are several neural pathways that have been extensively studied, which help researchers and physicians better understand the molecular underpinnings of memory.

These neural circuits involve several different key regions within the brain. The hippocampus is an integral member, but it is not the only structure involved (Fig. 1.12). The memory circuits within the brain are fairly complex, and also extremely sensitive. This sensitivity is classically thought to be one of the reasons why memory loss is one of the earliest symptoms of Alzheimer's disease, despite the presence of pathology in many other parts of the brain.

One interesting feature of this memory circuit, known as the Papez circuit, is the ubiquitous nature of the exact location in which memory formation takes place. The formation of a new memory begins in the hippocampus, but is propagated to various other parts of the brain, and the final memory is actually stored in several different parts of the brain, rather than a single discrete location. Imagine walking into a library to return a number of books you had checked out. The librarian that you first talk to in order to return the books can be thought of as the hippocampus. Once the books are returned, they are then placed back in their appropriate locations on bookshelves throughout the library. Thus, if each book was a small part of a single memory, then the memory as a whole is actually stored and spread out throughout the entire library. When that memory is to be recalled, several different locations of the brain (or library in the example) must be utilized in order to reform the memory. It might make sense that a particular memory is stored in a specific part of the brain — well, this is true to a degree; however, it is

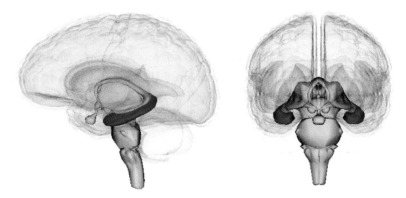

Fig. 1.12. The location of the hippocampus within the brain is highlighted. (Figure credit: Ref. 29.)

more accurate to think about different components of a single memory being stored in different anatomical locations within the brain. Thus, if a specific part of the cortex is damaged, it might affect only part of a memory, rather than destroying the entire memory.

This makes the treatment of Alzheimer's disease extremely difficult, since the failure of the memory system is a diffuse moving target and thus does not give scientists a discrete site to target drugs and therapies. As memories are formed, they must also be recalled. Therefore, there is a two-way street of memory encoding and retrieval that is always in play. Individuals who suffer from Alzheimer's disease experience difficulties in both memory encoding and recall. This manifests early on as transient memory gaps that initially resolve. For example, an individual with the earliest manifestations of Alzheimer's disease may forget the name of his or her grandchild, but they may be able to recall the name at some point of time in the future.

When one of the authors of this book used to conduct neuropsychological tests on patients with the earliest symptoms of Alzheimer's disease, the patients he tested would describe the feeling as a "tip-of-the-tongue" moment. This is the sensation in which they know what they want to say but they cannot find the right word, regardless of how hard they try. Many times, when they are no longer thinking about the word, it will pop back into their heads. Unfortunately, as the disease progresses, the ability to eventually recall the name disappears and the individual is left with a permanent loss of that memory. Alzheimer's disease has a relatively gradual onset — it does not just hit all of a sudden and cause drastic memory loss. Rather, it slowly and surely results in the deterioration of memory that evolves from mild problems to severe cognitive malfunctioning.

Studying the Brain

Since the brain is so well encapsulated by the skull and relatively difficult to manipulate, it is fairly arduous to study. One of the reasons that it is so challenging to study is that the product it produces, consciousness, is very difficult to quantify and analyze. Many of the earliest discoveries associating particular brain regions with specific cognitive functions were premised on linking discrete damage to the brain and the corresponding cognitive manifestations that ensued, thus enabling indirect

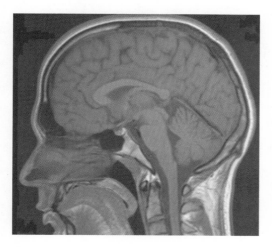

Fig. 1.13. A magnetic resonance imaging scan (MRI) of the brain. (Figure credit: Ref. 30.)

inferences about the function of that specific component of the brain. This method of determining brain function was replaced as new technologies emerged. One important technological advancement that made the study of the brain much more feasible was brain imaging.

Various imaging modalities such as magnetic resonance imaging (MRI) and computed axial tomography (CAT) scans — or CT scans — allow physicians and researchers to visualize the structural and functional components of the brain. Functional magnetic resource imaging (FMRI) even allows for the direct observation of the functional networks within the brain in real time. The development of these imaging tools led to a new chapter in neuroscience that resulted in a tremendously improved understanding of the human brain and how we can study it. Additionally, even more recent advances in brain imaging are allowing physicians to begin detecting Alzheimer's disease before

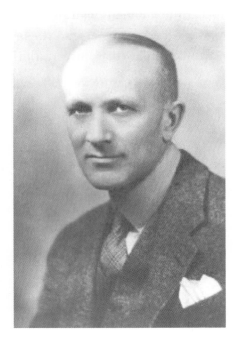

Fig. 1.14. Wilder Penfield began mapping the human brain during surgery. This helped elucidate the function of particular brain regions. (Figure credit: Ref. 31.)

patients exhibit clinically noticeable symptoms — we will expand on this in later chapters.

In addition to brain imaging, the various functions of discrete regions of the brain can also be studied intraoperatively. Beginning with Wilder Penfield, who published his work in 1951, neurological surgeons can use a probe with a small current passing through it to stimulate various parts of the brain. For example, by stimulating a specific part of the brain known as the motor cortex, a brain surgeon can evoke a physical response in the patient, such as making that patient's arm, leg, or body move once the electrical probe is placed on specific parts of the motor cortex. Penfield mapped parts of the cerebral cortex in order to identify the function of different parts of the human cortex. This direct approach to inferring brain function greatly contributed to the evolving field of neuroscience by connecting specific brain regions with their corresponding neurological functions.

Now that we have presented an overview of the human brain, its organization, its structure, and how we study it, we will explore what happens when the brain ages, and also when it becomes dysfunctional, as in the case of Alzheimer's disease.

References

1. Hartmann P, Ramseier A, Gudat F, *et al.* (1994) Normal weight of the brain in adults in relation to age, sex, body height and weight. Der *Pathologe* **15**(3): 165–170.
2. Willie CK, Smith KJ. (2011) Fuelling the exercising brain: A regulatory quagmire for lactate metabolism. *J Physiol* **589**(4): 779–780.
3. https://commons.wikimedia.org/wiki/Category:Brain#/media/File:AD_versus_CO.jpg
4. Agamanolis DP. (n.d.) *Cerebrospinal Fluid. Chapter 14.* [http://neuropathology-web.org/chapter14/chapter14CSF.html] [Accessed January 31, 2016].
5. https://commons.wikimedia.org/wiki/File:1317_CFS_Circulation.jpg
6. https://commons.wikimedia.org/wiki/Category:Cerebrospinal_fluid#/media/File:Dist_vent.png

7. http://physiologyonline.physiology.org/content/17/6/227
8. https://commons.wikimedia.org/wiki/File:Meninges-en.svg
9. Heber-Katz E, Stocum DL. (2013) *New Perspectives in Regeneration.* Springer.
10. Szymik B. (2011) A nervous journey. *ASU — Ask A Biologist.* [http://askabiologist.asu.edu/parts-nervous-system] [Accessed December 29, 2015].
11. The cells in your body. *Science NetLinks.* [http://sciencenetlinks.com/student-teacher-sheets/cells-your-body/] [Accessed January 31, 2016].
12. http://www.enchantedlearning.com/subjects/anatomy/brain/Neuron.shtml
13. https://en.wikipedia.org/wiki/Hair%27s_breadth
14. https://commons.wikimedia.org/wiki/File:1207_Neuron_Shape_Classification.jpg
15. http://cnx.org/contents/pMqJxKsZ@6/Nervous-System
16. https://upload.wikimedia.org/wikipedia/commons/a/a6/Blausen_0870_TypesofNeuroglia.png
17. https://commons.wikimedia.org/wiki/File:Neurons-axons-dendrites-synapses.PNG
18. Muckli L, Naumer MJ, Singer W. (2009) Bilateral visual field maps in a patient with only one hemisphere. *Proc Natl Acad Sci USA* **106**(31): 13034–13039.
19. http://www.bbc.com/news/health-31807961
20. http://www.parentfurther.com/ages-stages/3-5
21. http://www.psychology.emory.edu/cognition/rochat/Rochat5levels.pdf
22. https://en.wikipedia.org/wiki/Synaptic_pruning
23. https://en.wikipedia.org/wiki/Myelin
24. https://commons.wikimedia.org/wiki/Gyri#/media/File:PretermSurfaces_HiRes.png
25. Scheff SW, Price DA. (2006) Alzheimer's disease-related alterations in synaptic density: neocortex and hippocampus. *J Alzheimers Dis* **9**(3): 101–116.
26. https://commons.wikimedia.org/wiki/Category:Brain_lobes#/media/File:Blausen_0111_BrainLobes.png
27. http://www.human-memory.net/disorders_alzheimers.html
28. http://upload.wikimedia.org/wikipedia/commons/5/5b/Hippocampus_and_seahorse_cropped.JPG

29. https://commons.wikimedia.org/wiki/Category:Hippocampus_(anatomy)#/media/File:Hippocampus_image.png

30. https://commons.wikimedia.org/wiki/Magnetic_resonance_imaging#/media/File:Mrt_big.jpg

31. https://commons.wikimedia.org/wiki/Wilder_Penfield#/media/File:Wilder_Penfield.jpg

2 Dysfunction

"He had destroyed his talent by not using it, by betrayals of himself and what he believed in, by drinking so much that he blunted the edge of his perceptions, by laziness, by sloth, and by snobbery, by pride and by prejudice, by hook and by crook. What was this? A catalogue of old books? What was his talent anyway? It was a talent all right but instead of using it, he had traded on it. It was never what he had done, but always what he could do."

— *The Complete Short Stories of Ernest Hemingway* by Ernest Hemingway, Nobel Laureate (Literature, 1954)

The spectacular ability of the brain to remember, synthesize, and manipulate information makes it essential to the health and well-being of an individual. Yet amidst this spectacle, there are unfortunate opacities that illustrate just how the brain can malfunction, and how delicately beautiful it really is. Unfortunately, there are many different things that can harm the brain, ranging from environmental insults such as alcohol, to trauma and neurodegenerative disorders such as Alzheimer's or Parkinson's disease (PD).

When things begin to go wrong within the brain, they are sometimes difficult to detect. The reason for this is the incredible amount of redundancy and overlap within the brain itself. Initially, as specific cognitive functions begin to deteriorate, they are so well protected that the problems are usually masked until the abnormal process progresses to a later stage. This is readily seen in children, who are notorious within the medical community for their ability to compensate for prolonged periods of time and then deteriorate precipitiously and usually irreversibly in many medical and trauma scenarios. This is because children can compensate against shock, which is an inability to maintain normal blood pressure, much better than adults. Children can maintain a normal blood pressure after losing up to 30% of their blood volume, while adults show signs of shock after only a 10% loss.[1] Children will therefore deteriorate slowly and then decompensate quickly, while adults have a gradual decline prior to decompensation. These changes are in part due to significant differences in bodily systems, body size, and blood volume. Therefore, the early detection of shock in children is a critical component of the proper provision of healthcare. Similarly, early detection of abnormalities in the brain is critically important for preventing and treating serious medical disorders. The early detection of disease allows physicians to recognize a problem and initiate preventative therapies in order to delay the onset of the disease, or even thwart the damaging effects of the disease altogether.

In the fight to eradicate Alzheimer's disease, many different factors, including that of early detection, must be understood and effectively implemented. The challenges in early detection, however, have prevented scientists and doctors from identifying pathology in patients until it is far too late. Unlike diabetes, which can be readily monitored and diagnosed with a simple blood sample, or an infection that can be cultured or identified with a laboratory test, Alzheimer's disease does not have a readily accessible marker that can help in its identification. This makes it a particularly challenging disease to study, and even more challenging to treat.

Normal Age-related Changes

As individuals age, there are certain expected changes that are normal aspects of aging. These changes are the result of years of use. The human body, just like any structure in the universe, is prone to the trials and damages of time. There are many factors that lead to the normal degeneration of the human body with age. One important factor is the accumulation of genetic mutations over the course of an individual's lifetime. These mutations can lead to varying degrees of changes within the cell. Some mutations might alter the cell's ability to grow and regenerate itself, while other mutations can be completely neutral and result in no significant deleterious changes in the cell.

If the mutations are too damaging, the cell has several options. The first option is to undergo pre-programmed cell death, or apoptosis. This prevents the cell from negatively affecting its neighboring cells, and also prevents it from becoming cancerous. In fact, anytime a cell is sufficiently damaged, apoptosis occurs. Apoptosis is a complex pre-programmed process that involves the specific activation of genes that lead to the synthesis of the proteins or enzymes that carry out this process. As abnormal proteins that form plaques and tangles accumulate within the brain in Alzheimer's disease, neurons that are exposed to these toxic proteins eventually undergo apoptosis and commit cellular suicide. This is one of the ways in which the brain changes in Alzheimer's disease. In fact, this cell death causes the brain to shrink — otherwise known as atrophy — as a whole in Alzheimer's disease.

Besides apoptosis, DNA damage can lead to another less desirable complication: cancer. As cells accumulate various mutations in their genome, they may begin moving down the cancer pipeline. Cancer, in a nutshell, is the uncontrolled growth and proliferation of cells. If the molecular pathways that normally serve to control the growth rate, the ability to spread and invade through tissue, and the cell's ability to undergo apoptosis are damaged or nonfunctional, then that cell may grow uncontrollably and invade into other parts of the body. This is an unfortunate consequence of DNA damage due to mutations that accumulate over time, and is why cancer rates are so prevalent in older individuals.

In addition to apoptosis and cancer, DNA mutations can also cause a cell to fall into a middle ground, in which it is not functioning at its optimum, but is still functional enough not to undergo apoptosis or be cancerous. In this state, a cell can serve its normal functions, but to a diminished degree. Thus, if a cell that normally ensures that neurons have a healthy environment in which to live is damaged and cannot execute its functions perfectly, the neurons it supports may be altered and thus be more prone to damage.

Another example of why individuals exhibit normal changes with aging is due to the shortening of the protective regions found at the ends of DNA, known as telomeres. Telomeres are long stretches of DNA that are found on the ends of chromosomes. When chromosomes replicate in normal cell division, the ends of the chromosomes become shortened. Thus, the telomeres, which do not necessarily produce any significant gene products, are shortened instead of regions of DNA that are critical to normal cell functions. Imagine a book, and every time we opened this book, the first and last page fell off. Well this is directly analogous to chromosomes — every time a chromosome replicates, a small bit of the beginning and end of the chromosome is lost. If we were to add hundreds of blanks pages at the beginning and the end of a book, the blank pages would be the ones that were lost every time we opened the book, and thus the important contents of the book would be preserved and protected. This is what the telomeres basically function to do — protect important parts of DNA from being damaged during normal cell replication (Fig. 2.1).

The issue that arises, however, is that as we age, our telomeres shorten. There is actually a cellular process that is carried out by an enzyme known as telomerase that functions to extend the telomeres at the ends of chromosomes. Despite the functions of telomerase, the telomeres continue to shrink, and once they are completely gone, the important parts of DNA will then be destroyed as the cell replicates. Thus, as we age, we will eventually reach a critical threshold in which our telomeres are too short to serve in their protective roles, and we will begin to damage critical parts of our DNA. This further leads to cellular damage, and eventually contributes to "normal" age-related changes.

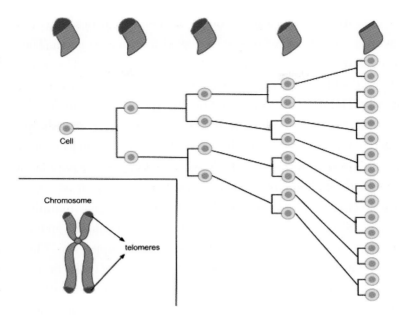

Fig. 2.1.   Shortening of telomeres (shown in red) with cellular division. As cells divide, the telomeres (which protect the ends of DNA) are progressively shortened. At a certain point, known as the Hayflick limit, cellular division can lead to the destruction of DNA and may contribute to natural aging. After approximately 40–60 replications, the cell will usually undergo apoptosis, or programmed cell death.[2] (Figure credit: Ref. 3.)

In addition to cellular changes, physical and mental age-related changes can also be seen in individuals. Some of the standard physical changes associated with age include changes in skin, hair, height, weight, vision, sleep, and hearing. Skin becomes less elastic and more wrinkled due to a loss of collagen, fingernail growth slows, and oil glands decrease in function and cause drier skin (these changes can be modified by using moisturizer and sunscreen, as well as mitigating sun exposure to skin). Hair can become thinner, more brittle, and will lose pigment, resulting in grayness. Even height decreases with age — individuals can lose up to 2 inches of height by age 80, due to loss of bone density, changes in body posture and compression of the vertebrae, joints, and intervertebral disks.

One study was conducted on 8,003 men of Japanese ancestry with an average age of 54, who were followed for over 40 years. The study investigated the effects of height on aging and longevity.[4] The researchers analyzed the effects of height and a particular gene, known as *FOXO3*, on longevity. The results showed that height, specifically in middle life, has a positive association with mortality. It was determined that shorter stature actually predicts a longer life span. In fact, individuals shorter than 158 cm (5 feet 2 inches) had the longest life span in the population that was studied. Additionally, it was determined that height was associated with a specific gene, known as the *FOXO3* gene. This gene is implicated in the regulation of normal fasting levels of insulin, and may be an important regulator of health and also function as a tumor suppressor. Therefore, the association between height and longevity may actually be mediated by the *FOXO3* genotype and could be the reason why shorter height was associated with a longer life span. This is an interesting study that serves to reflect the fact that certain unchangeable physical and genetic characteristics may play a role in longevity. However, there are many modifiable risk factors that can also dramatically influence longevity.

In addition to the variety of physical changes that are commonly associated with aging, individuals are also prone to developing sensory changes as they age. One of the most common senses to be affected by age is the sense of hearing. High-frequency sounds become more difficult to hear and tone perception diminishes. Vision is also affected, with the most common change being difficulty reading text — this is due to the lenses in the eyes becoming less flexible (*presbyopia*). Night vision and visual acuity (sharpness) also deteriorates with age. Age-related macular degeneration (AMD) is also very common with age, and is a common cause of blindness in individuals older than 50 years of age.[5]

Smell

One sensory change that has actually been heavily implicated in dementia is the sense of smell (olfaction). In fact, one component of a thorough neurological examination is the assessment of olfaction. Diagnosing Alzheimer's disease prior to the development of clinical symptoms is very difficult. Doctors traditionally monitor for signs of the neurodegenerative disease by performing a series of extensive tests in order to analyze the patient's cognitive functions. However, recent studies have highlighted an alternative method that suggests that our sense of smell could be used to diagnose Alzheimer's disease. Studies have found that an impaired sense of smell is one of the earliest symptoms of Alzheimer's, Parkinson's, and other neurodegenerative diseases. In fact, implementing something as simple as a scratch-and-sniff smell test could become a cheaper and faster way for doctors to detect signs of traumatic brain injury (*TBI*) and neurodegenerative ailments.

Jennifer Stamps from the University of Florida's McKnight Brain Institute Center conducted a series of experiments suggesting that scent and Alzheimer's disease are related. During her study, 94 participants with varying causes of neurodegenerative diseases, including Alzheimer's disease, were blindfolded and tested for their ability to detect an odor, one nostril at a time.[6] The researchers at this institute used a small container of peanut butter held at the bottom of a ruler to measure the distance from each nostril. When the participants exhaled, the researcher moved the container up by 1 cm until the person was able to detect the odor. Upon odor detection, the distance between the subject's nostril and the container was measured.

Interestingly, the results of this study suggest that individuals with Alzheimer's disease had a more difficult time detecting the odor while using their left nostril when compared to their right nostril. In order to better understand the significance of these results, a region in the brain called the temporal lobe, which houses the primary parts of the brain associated with smelling (olfaction) and hearing (audition), was studied. The two temporal lobes function in interpreting auditory and olfactory sensations. Smell, unlike sight, is ipsilateral, meaning that the side of the body sensing the stimulus and the side of the brain processing the information are the same.[7] The study that was conducted using peanut butter on the test subjects underscored the notion that portions of the olfactory smell complex are the initial sites of Alzheimer's disease pathology and that patients with Alzheimer's disease often have more degeneration of their left than right hemisphere. Naturally, the number of olfactory receptor cells declines with age; however, subjects with lower scores on a smell test are more likely to show frontal lobe damage during brain imaging than those whose sense of smell is normal.[8]

Another approach to olfactory testing came from psychiatrist Davangere Devanand of Columbia University, who noted that smell is the first sense to be affected by Alzheimer's, with the hallmark protein tangles of Alzheimer's disease appearing early in the olfactory bulb. Devanand and his colleagues conducted a study by looking at the results of multiple-choice scratch-and-sniff tests in which 1,037 older individuals were asked to recognize 40 scents. The results indicated that lower scores on the multiple-choice tests can accurately predict cognitive decline and are associated with increased rates of dementia. In fact, they found that for each point missed on the test, the risk of developing dementia rose by 10%. Furthermore, lower initial scores on the multiple-choice scratch-and-sniff test were significantly associated with cognitive decline.

The deterioration of an individual's sense of smell could result from a variety of intermingling factors, including damage due to TBI. Hyposmia, a condition associated with TBI in which the individual's ability to smell or detect odors is diminished, can even be confirmed by olfactory testing.[9] Ultimately, patients suffering from such cases of olfactory deterioration are at risk of developing Alzheimer's disease. Olfactory loss is not only an early warning sign of Alzheimer's disease, but also of several other neurological disorders. One study published in 1999 by Amy Bornstein Graves at the University of South Florida investigated senior citizens with no signs of dementia. The study found that individuals with no sense of smell and who also had the *APOE-e4* allele (a genetic risk factor for Alzheimer's disease) had a five-times greater likelihood of developing cognitive decline than individuals with normal smell and no

APOE-e4 allele.[10] Furthermore, a study conducted at Harvard Medical School administered the same 40-item smell test to healthy older adults. This study showed that individuals with a lesser ability to identify scents had smaller brain volumes in two critical areas associated with memory (known as the entorhinal cortex and the hippocampus), and also were more likely to have worse memory than adults with a normal sense of smell.[11]

Finally, a series of olfactory or scratch-and-sniff tests can be used by doctors to prevent a misdiagnosis. Diseases such as depression are often misdiagnosed as Alzheimer's disease PD; however, they are accompanied by little or no smell loss. In such cases, olfactory testing can be useful to differentiate disorders and to ensure a correct diagnosis.

These sensory changes can be extremely problematic as people age, especially when they increase the risk of falls and accidents in elderly individuals. In addition to the physical and sensory changes that regularly accompany aging, sleep can also unfortunately be adversely affected by age. As we get older, the circadian rhythm that normally regulates our sleep cycle and the various stages of sleep is modified. This leads to fewer total hours of sleep in general and shallower stages of sleep, and thwarts the normal homeostatic role that sleep serves.

Sleep is an incredibly important aspect of normal health, and has even been implicated in Alzheimer's disease. A recent study showed that sleep plays a critical role in the elimination of toxins, such as β-amyloid from the brain.[12,13] This study supported the idea that sleep serves a critical function, which is not surprising, since sleep is a conserved trait of all animal species. The study conducted at the University of Rochester and New York University found that sleep is crucial to maintaining metabolic homeostasis in the brain. When individuals are asleep or, interestingly, anesthetized, the amount of fluid-filled space surrounding the neurons in the brain (known as the interstitial space) decreases by 60%. This decreases the interplay of cerebrospinal fluid (CSF) with interstitial fluid, which in turn decreases the clearance of β-amyloid from the brain. β-amyloid is a hallmark of Alzheimer's disease and is an abnormal protein that forms senile plaques within the brains of Alzheimer's patients. Additionally, the amount of CSF produced differs in the sleep and wakeful state, with increased production during sleep. This suggests that sleep is an extremely important function that helps remove toxic components from the brain and may play an important role in the development of Alzheimer's disease.

Nervous System Damage and Neurogenesis

Damage to either the peripheral nervous system (*PNS*) or central nervous system (*CNS*), whether from trauma or a neurodegenerative diseases such as Alzheimer's, usually results in an inability of nerve cells to transmit signals, thus causing loss of function in the afflicted person. Originally, this neuronal damage — mild or severe — was thought to be permanent and irreversible. Although typical cellular regeneration (mitotic division) of the supportive glial cells had been previously observed, neuroscientists and neurologists, including Nobel Laureate and father of modern neuroscience Santiago Ramón y Cajal, considered neurons to be sentient and incapable of regeneration.[14,15] Essentially, early neuroscientists believed that individuals are born with a distinct number of neurons, a number that could only remain the same or decrease throughout one's life. The idea that we only get a set number of neurons was first contested in 1962, but it was not until the 1980s that the scientific community began to realize that not only are mammals capable of fixing damaged neurons, but also mammalian brains are continually regenerating new neurons through a process called "neurogenesis."[16,17]

Recent research shows that mammals, including humans, have the capability to restore functionality after neurodegeneration. Although our regenerative capabilities are limited, we can either regrow the specific portions of the neurons that were damaged or undergo neurogenesis in order to generate completely new neurons to replace those that have been lost. Unfortunately, restoring damaged neurons is more successfully executed in the PNS than in the brain or the spinal cord. This disparity in nervous system regeneration depends on a few factors, but is mainly due to the types of glial cells available within the CNS or PNS.[18] A Schwann cell is a specific type of glial cell that creates an insulating sheath around the neurons of the PNS (a process called "myelination") in order to protect and aid those neurons. Interestingly, they also produce a multitude of proteins that create a path for and significantly aid the regeneration of a damaged neuron.[19–22]

Unlike the neurons in the PNS, the neurons in the CNS are myelinated by another type of glial cell called "oligodendrocytes." Oligodendrocytes are not as versatile as Schwann cells and therefore do not promote neural regeneration as well.[23–25] However, the brain has its own mechanism of neurogenesis to partially make up for the lack of neuronal repair in the CNS. During adulthood, the development of new neurons is initiated from neural stem cells (stem cells that can only turn into neurons) in two regions of the brain: the *subventricular zone.* (see Fig. 2.2) and the *subgranular zone*.

These adult neural stem cells first form into neuroblasts, which are essentially immature preliminary neurons. Neuroblasts then mature with time, and stay in the subgranular zone or subventricular zone, or they travel to the *olfactory bulb (OB)* via the *rostral migratory stream (RMS)*(see Fig. 2.3).

Neurogenesis in Alzheimer's and Brain Tumors

Most important to Alzheimer's disease is neurogenesis occurring in the SGZ, for the SGZ is within the area of the brain that is associated with memory and learning (the hippocampus). In fact, studies in mice have linked Alzheimer's disease to decreased neurogenesis within the SGZ.[27] Furthermore, regulatory molecules found during SGZ neurogenesis have been investigated as potential therapies for Alzheimer's disease in order to increase neurogenesis and replace dying neurons faster.[28,29]

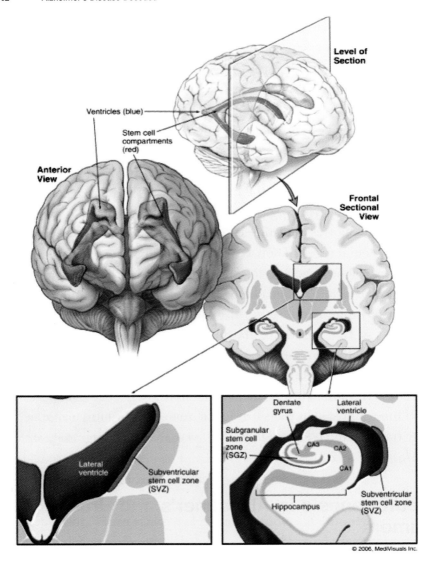

Fig. 2.2.   The subventricular zone (SVZ) can be found in the bottom-left picture and in the bottom-right picture underneath the *lateral ventricles* in the top picture. The subgranular zone (SGZ) can be found underneath the dentate gyrus within the hippocampus in the bottom-right picture. (Figure credit: Image obtained from MediVisuals, Inc.)

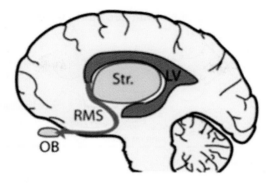

Fig. 2.3. The rostral migratory stream (RMS) is shown with a red line in the right half of the brain that is depicted. The RMS allows for the migration of neuroblasts from the subventricular zone at the end of the lateral ventricle (LV) to the olfactory bulb (OB), where they can mature into neurons. (Figure credit: Ref. 26.)

It is important to note that neurogenesis is inherently different from other forms of cellular regeneration. Neurogenesis is most similar to stem cells differentiating into a new cell, as opposed to other forms of tissue regeneration, which are performed by cellular division (known as mitotic division). Mitotic division has been described as "an intricate chemical dance that's part individual, part community driven," meaning that not only does it depend on the mechanisms within each cell, but also the available space, nutrients, and permission for growth.[30] In this process, also known as mitosis, each cell must replicate all of its genetic blueprints (DNA) in order to form two new cells that are identical to each other. After a few rounds of replication, the cells typically stop regenerating either due to limited space and nutrients, the presence of stop-signaling molecules, or both.

Unfortunately, mitosis is far from perfect, and errors resulting in mutations are easily made during the replication process. Several fail-safes and regulatory mechanisms exist within the body in order to protect against random mutations by destroying improperly replicated cells, although some mutated cells manage to bypass the fail-safes and remain within the body. If enough mutations occur within a given cell, then that cell can become cancerous and completely ignore the limitations of

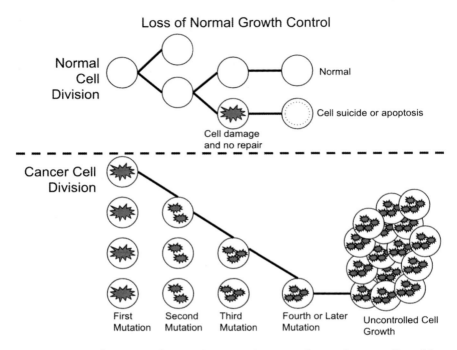

Fig. 2.4. Regular mitotic division (top image) is imperfect, and eventually yields a mutated cell. If the mutation is noticed, then the cell dies by suicide or is killed by the immune system. However, if the cell goes by unnoticed and multiple other mutations occur (bottom image) through more rounds of replication, then the cell will become cancerous and divide uncontrollably.

space, nutrients, or stop-signaling molecules and continually divide to form a tumor (see Fig. 2.4). This stepwise process of tumor formation is the same in all types of tissue, whether it is the skin, muscular tissue, skeletal tissue, or nervous tissue. Therefore, because neurogenesis is an inherently different process from mitotic replication and glial cells alone undergo mitosis, most brain tumors tend to be of glial origin and are known as gliomas.

Although there is a lot that can go wrong with the brain and the human body, especially as we age, a long and healthy life can still be observed in many individuals. However, one thing that is extremely important to keep in mind is that normal healthy aging should be devoid of any abnormal disease processes such as cancer, heart disease, and Alzheimer's disease. Normal aging does not always entail memory loss, disease, and hardships, but rather can be filled with fulfillment, health, exercise, and meaningful life experiences with friends and family. We will explore normal aging and the misconception of senility being a part of normal aging in the next chapter.

References

1. http://centegra.org/wp-content/uploads/2013/06/Pediatric-Trauma.pdf
2. Shay JW, Wright WE. (2000) Hayflick, his limit, and cellular ageing. *Nat Rev Mol Cell Biol* **1**(1): 72–76.
3. https://upload.wikimedia.org/wikipedia/commons/7/72/Hayflick_Limit_%281%29.svg
4. He QM, Morris BJ, Grove JS, *et al.* (2014) Shorter men live longer: Association of height with longevity and *FOXO3* genotype in American men of Japanese ancestry. *PLoS One* **9**(5): e94385.
5. Facts about age-related macular degeneration. [https://nei.nih.gov/health/maculardegen/armd_facts] [Accessed January 31, 2016].
6. Stamps, JJ, Bartoshuk LM, Heilman KM. (2013) A brief olfactory test for Alzheimer's disease. *J Neurol Sci* **333**(1): 19–24.
7. http://www.npr.org/sections/health-shots/2013/10/11/232135483/why-a-peanut-butter-test-for-alzheimers-might-be-too-simple
8. http://www.scientificamerican.com/article/smell-tests-could-one-day-reveal-head-trauma-and-neurodegenerative-disease/
9. http://www.the-scientist.com/?articles.view/articleNo/37603/title/Smell-and-the-Degenerating-Brain/
10. Graves AB, Bowen JD, Rajaram L, *et al.* (1999) Impaired olfaction as a marker for cognitive decline: Interaction with apolipoprotein E epsilon4 status. *Neurology* **53**: 1480–1487.
11. https://www.alzheimers.org.uk/site/scripts/press_article.php?pressReleaseID=1154
12. Mendelsohn AR, Larrick JW. (2013) Sleep facilitates clearance of metabolites from the brain: Glymphatic function in aging and neurodegenerative diseases. *Rejuvenation Res* **16**(6): 518–523.

13. Xie L, Kang H, Xu Q, *et al.* (2013) Sleep drives metabolite clearance from the adult brain. *Science* **342**(6156): 373–377.

14. Altman J. (1962) Are new neurons formed in the brains of adult mammals? *Science* **135**(3509): 1127–1128.

15. Mandal A. (2010) What is neurogenesis? *News-Medical.net*. AZoNetwork. [http://www.news-medical.net/health/What-is-Neurogenesis.aspx] [Accessed December 29, 2015].

16. Bayer SA, Yackel JW, Puri PS. (1982) Neurons in the rat dentate gyrus granular layer substantially increase during juvenile and adult life. *Science* **216**(4548): 890–892.

17. Goldman SA, Nottebohm F. (1983) Neuronal production, migration, and differentiation in a vocal control nucleus of the adult female canary brain. *Proc Natl Acad Sci USA* **80**(8): 2390–2394.

18. Huebner EA, Strittmatter SM. (2009) Axon regeneration in the peripheral and central nervous systems. *Results Probl Cell Differ* **48**: 339–351.

19. Bailey SB, Eichler ME, Villadiego A, Rich KM. (1993) The influence of fibronectin and laminin during Schwann cell migration and peripheral nerve regeneration through silicon chambers. *J Neurocytol* **22**(3): 176–184.

20. Frostick SP, Yin Q, Kemp GJ. (1998) Schwann cells, neurotrophic factors, and peripheral nerve regeneration. *Microsurgery* **18**(7): 397–405.

21. Terenghi G. (1999) Peripheral nerve regeneration and neurotrophic factors. *J Anat* **194**(1): 1–14.

22. Thornton MR, Mantovani C, Birchall MA, Terenghi G. (2005) Quantification of N-CAM and N-cadherin expression in axotomized and crushed rat sciatic nerve. *J Anat* **206**(1): 69–78.

23. Fawcett JW, Asher RA. (1999) The glial scar and central nervous system repair. *Brain Res Bull* **49**(6): 377–391.

24. Fawcett JW. (2006) Overcoming inhibition in the damaged spinal cord. *J Neurotrauma* **23**(3–4): 371–383.

25. Yiu G, He ZG. (2006) Glial inhibition of CNS axon regeneration. *Nat Rev Neurosci* **7**(8): 617–627.

26. van Strien ME, van den Berge SA, Hol EM. (2011) Migrating neuroblasts in the adult human brain: A stream reduced to a trickle. *Cell Res* **21**(11): 1523.

27. Marx CE, Trost WT, Shampine LJ, *et al.* (2006) The neurosteroid allopregnanolone is reduced in prefrontal cortex in Alzheimer's disease. *Biol Psychiatry* **60**(12): 1287–1294.

28. Mu YL, Gage FH. (2011) Adult hippocampal neurogenesis and its role in Alzheimer's disease. *Mol Neurodegener* **6**(1): 85.

29. Cissé M, Checler F. (2015) Eph receptors: New players in Alzheimer's disease pathogenesis. *Neurobiol Dis* **73**: 137–149.

30. Zaidan G. (2012) How do cancer cells behave differently from healthy ones? *YouTube.* [https://www.youtube.com/watch?v=BmFEoCFDi-w] [Accessed December 29, 2015].

Chapter 3

Senility and Normal Aging

"Worry never robs tomorrow of its sorrow, it only saps today of its joy."

— Leo Buscaglia, American author and motivational speaker

Is Alzheimer's Disease a Normal Part of Aging?

It has become relatively common to associate memory loss and senility with the normal aging process. This is an incorrect association that is undoubtedly present due to the high frequency of dementia in the aging population.

It is very important to understand that Alzheimer's disease and any other cause of dementia are not normal processes associated with aging. Rather, they are abnormal processes. This can be illustrated by thinking about diabetes, which is generally thought of as an abnormal disease process. Well, diabetes (specifically Type II diabetes) occurs when the body builds up a tolerance to insulin (a protein that allows sugar to enter the body's cells). This generally occurs when individuals have unhealthy diets, and occurs frequently in individuals who are obese. However, the development of diabetes is not normal, despite the fact that it occurs relatively commonly in individuals who have poor diets and frequently are obese.

This is similar to Alzheimer's disease. As individuals age, their bodies change in various ways. However, normal healthy aging results in slow changes that really do not significantly limit the productivity of senior citizens. In fact, many people have studied the health of individuals in their ninth and tenth and decades of life and found that these people can be extremely healthy and fit. In fact, if individuals did not die of heart disease, cancer, Alzheimer's disease, and other common causes of death, they would likely live into their tenth decade of life in a healthy and productive fashion.

An ongoing study known as the "90+ Study" is being conducted at the University of California Irvine. It is led by Dr. Claudia Kawas and began in 2003. Its purpose is to study individuals who are 90 years of age and older who, interestingly enough, are the fastest growing age group in the US. Over 1,600 people are being followed and are receiving neurological and psychological tests every 6 months. Information on the participants' diet, activities, and medical health are obtained, in addition to a battery of cognitive and physical tests to look at the participants' well-being. The 90+ Study seeks to determine what factors are associated with longer lives, to understand cognitive decline and clinical changes, and to gather epidemiological data on individuals who are over 90 years old.

The published findings of the 90+ Study have been extremely interesting and informative. Researchers have found that individuals who drink moderate amounts of alcohol or coffee live longer than those who do not drink any. The reasons for this are unclear; however, the antioxidants found in red wine and coffee, as well as the psychological changes associated with both drinks, may play a contributory role.[1] Additionally, individuals "who were overweight in their 70s lived longer than normal or underweight people did." Again, the reason for this is unclear; however, other studies have found that being overweight in middle age is also protective against the development of dementia.[2] The 90+ Study also found that "over 40% of people aged 90 and older suffer from dementia while almost 80% are disabled." This was true in women more so than men. Interestingly, half of the individuals who are over 90 years of age with dementia do not have any neuropathological changes in their brain that correlate with or explain their cognitive changes. Another finding of the study that directly relates to Alzheimer's disease is that individuals who are over 90 years of age and who have the *APOE-e2* gene are less likely to develop Alzheimer's disease. However, these same individuals are also more likely to have Alzheimer's neuropathology in their brains. This is an extremely interesting finding that adds to the difficulties of understanding the disease process and being able to predict which individuals will develop Alzheimer's disease and which will not.

Thus, Alzheimer's disease interferes with the normal process of healthy aging and alters the trajectory in an unfavorable fashion. It drastically shortens the afflicted individual's life expectancy, dampens the individual's productivity, diminishes the individual's cognitive capacity, and deteriorates the quality of life of the affected individual and their family. This is an unfortunate and far too common pathological process that destroys the joy and happiness that are normally associated with retirement and the later decades of life.

Despite its prevalence as individuals age, Alzheimer's disease is not normal and should not be an expected part of aging. The prevalence of Alzheimer's disease sharply increases as individuals age. Commonly, the age normally associated with an increased risk of Alzheimer's disease is 65. In fact, after the age of 65, the risk of developing Alzheimer's disease doubles every 5 years.[3] This is a shocking statistic and serves to address why Alzheimer's disease is so ubiquitously associated with old age and is sometimes considered a normal part of aging, when in fact it is not. As nation states begin to learn more about Alzheimer's disease and come to realize that it is in fact an abnormal disease process that should not be occurring, we may begin to focus more effort and dedicate more resources to better understanding the disease process itself and, more importantly, how it can be modified, prevented, or cured.

Where did the Term "Senility" Come From and Why is it Ubiquitously Associated with Aging?

The term "senile" originates from the mid-17th century, from the French word *sénile* and the Latin word *senilis*, which mean "old man."

The colloquial meaning of the term has evolved over the years, however, and senile has almost become a derogatory term to represent the proverbial "crazy, forgetful, delirious" old man who talks to himself. This is an unfortunate connotation that highlights the social and medical challenges that individuals with dementia face. Senility has become ubiquitously associated with old age, limiting the consideration that the confusion, memory loss, personality changes, and cognitive decline commonly associated with aging are actually due to an abnormal underlying disease process, rather than a representation of normal aging.

An individual can be construed as "senile" for a variety of reasons — most commonly due to dementia. However, other psychiatric and neurological disorders, such as schizophrenia, bipolar disorder, depression, or Parkinson's disease (PD), may also lead to an interpretation of senility. Normally, senility and aging should not be grouped together in the natural healthy aging process, but since Alzheimer's disease is such a prevalent part of aging, and due to the fact that it leads to the phenotype commonly construed as senile, the two terms have become nearly synonymous.

Generations from now, once a treatment for Alzheimer's disease has proven successful and dramatically decreased the presence of the disease, senility will no longer be considered a normal part of the aging process. Rather, it will be seen as an abnormal disease entity that is separate from the normal aging process and should be viewed as a disease that warrants early diagnosis, intervention, and treatment.

Cognitive Reserve

As any disease process manifests itself in the brain, there is a cushioning window such that the brain is able to resist damage. This cushioning window sometimes obscures any underlying problems until the resiliency of the brain is overcome and the disease overtly manifests itself — usually at a point where preventative treatment is no longer an option.

One of the best ways to mitigate the damaging effects of Alzheimer's disease is by extending the cushioning window. This can be accomplished by increasing the number of connections between the neurons within the brain. It is rather intuitive — a brain with more connections will be able to resist a disease that causes neuronal connections to be destroyed for a longer period of time than a brain with fewer connections. These neuronal — or synaptic — connections can be increased in a multitude of ways. Although a major predictor of the density of synaptic connections is inherently genetic, there are several environmental factors that can influence synaptic density.

One of these environmental factors is education. Education and lifelong learning promote the creation and strengthening of new and existing synaptic connections. Although there is a tangible limit to the degree with which education can protect against the development of Alzheimer's disease, the robust neuronal networks that evolve as a consequence of education undoubtedly ward off the devastating effects of the disease process to some degree.

Similarly, there is strong epidemiological evidence published in multiple journals that bilingualism, or speaking two languages, delays the onset of Alzheimer's disease.[4] This idea that education protects against Alzheimer's disease falls within the concept of cognitive reserve. The concept of cognitive reserve was initially proposed by Stern, and states that factors such as diet, education, occupation, exercise, and less stress, can increase an individual's ability to resist damage to the brain.[5] Scientists believe that education and learning (as well as a healthy diet and exercise) leads to an increase in cognitive reserve by way of establishing more synapses and networks in the brain. This causes the brain to be more resilient against neurological damage; in other words, this is a form of compensation against β-amyloid and the other pathologies of Alzheimer's.

By the same token, there are Nobel Prize-winning scientists who succumb to Alzheimer's disease at the same age as individuals who never completed their primary school education.[6] Thus, it is extremely difficult to predict which individuals will be affected by Alzheimer's disease and how the disease process will manifest itself. Some individuals are able

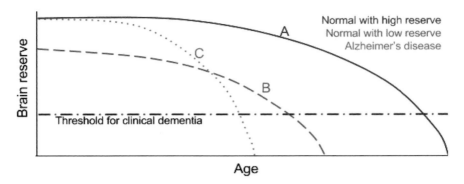

Fig. 3.1.   Line A depicts normal healthy individuals as they age. Line B depicts individuals with less cognitive reserve as they age. Line C depicts individuals with Alzheimer's disease. (Modified from Ref. 9.)

to survive many years after the diagnosis of Alzheimer's disease, while others survive only 2 years. This may be in part because of differences in age at diagnosis and the stage of the disease at diagnosis; however, there is certainly a great degree of heterogeneity in how individuals progress once they are diagnosed with Alzheimer's disease. On average, individuals live for a period of 8–10 years after the diagnosis of Alzheimer's disease (Fig. 3.1).[7]

Alzheimer's disease unfortunately destroys critical neural pathways in the brain, and eventually leads to severe cognitive decline to the point of a vegetative state, and eventually death. Although education can help deter the onset of the earliest cognitive symptoms, it eventually yields to the damaging effects of the disease process. Fortunately, there are several other environmental factors that can help delay the onset of Alzheimer's disease.

There is a commonly held belief that if you are an active lifelong learner and keep your brain engaged in various mental exercises, you could ward off Alzheimer's disease. This is an interesting notion that is somewhat grounded in science, but altogether unclear. The scientific principle that the belief is referring to is cognitive reserve. Let us put it this way: if you want to build the world's largest skyscraper, you want to incorporate built-in redundancies that help bolster and support the strength of the skyscraper. That way, if there is some sort of natural disaster, such as an earthquake, the building will have extra support and strength that may prevent it from toppling. However, given a big enough earthquake, the building will fall. This is analogous to Alzheimer's disease. Throughout an individual's life, he or she can increase the number of connections — or synapses — made between the neurons in their brain (known scientifically as increased synaptic density). This increase in synaptic density acts like the reinforcements to the building and helps ward off any underlying disease process, since there are simply more connections that must be destroyed before clinical symptoms become manifest.

Thus, an individual who is cognitively active, always learning, and always integrating new information will live a longer period of time before having clinically significant symptoms, such as memory loss, than a similar individual who lived a sedentary and cognitively unstimulating lifestyle. However, as the disease progresses, the clinical symptoms will undoubtedly manifest and untangle the years of experience, memories, and cognitive capacity of that individual's mind.

Several patients whom we have seen over the years have asked me what sorts of things are associated with an increase in cognitive reserve. Interestingly, it is multifactorial. One component is academic. For example, the number of years an individual has been in school, the type of education and training that individual has gone through, and whether or not they are lifelong learners and continue to take classes and attempt to learn new things throughout their life are all factors that contribute to the degree of synaptic density within the brain. These factors may also allow individuals who are cognitively more adept to be able to better compensate for the deficits associated with Alzheimer's disease. Additionally, these factors have all been shown to be correlated with a delayed onset of Alzheimer's disease. Another factor that has been shown to be protective with regards to the development of Alzheimer's disease is social activity. Individuals with diverse and complicated social networks, such as those who have large integrated families, a large network of friends, and individuals who socially interact with many people on a frequent basis, also develop Alzheimer's disease on average later than their less socially active peers.[8]

Other factors that contribute to the onset of Alzheimer's disease include things such as optimism and cardiovascular health. In general, things that are beneficial to the brain (lifelong learning, decreased levels of stress, and not having heart disease) help prevent against Alzheimer's disease, while things that are toxic to the brain (drinking, having increased cortisol levels related to stress, poor cardiovascular health, or living a sedentary lifestyle) increase the risk of developing Alzheimer's disease.

Thus, any effort that will be made to comprehensively treat Alzheimer's disease in the future must take into account the multifactorial nature of the pathological progression of the disease, and must urge patients to adopt lifelong habits that are good for their brains. This again is analogous to the recommendations made by physicians to individuals with cardiovascular disease or who are at risk of developing it. When a doctor orders a blood test and finds that the patient is at increased risk for developing heart disease, one of the first things that is recommended, along with medication, is a change in diet, exercise, and the lifestyle of the patient. This addresses the many other contributing factors of heart disease and is much more effective at preventing the onset of the disease than medication alone. A similar approach must be adopted for Alzheimer's disease and dementia. But what exactly is dementia, and how does Alzheimer's disease relate to it?

References

1. http://www.huffingtonpost.com/2013/10/17/coffee-health-benefits_n_4102133.html
2. https://www.washingtonpost.com/world/new-research-being-fat-in-middle-age-cuts-risk-of-developing-dementia/2015/04/10/c87512ec-df52-11e4-a1b8-2ed88bc190d2_story.html

3. http://www.nia.nih.gov/alzheimers/publication/preventing-alzheimers-disease/risk-factors-alzheimers-disease

4. Craik FIM, Bialystok E, Freedman M. (2010) Delaying the onset of Alzheimer disease: Bilingualism as a form of cognitive reserve. *Neurology* **75**(19): 1726–1729.

5. Stern Y. (2009) Cognitive reserve. *Neuropsychologia* **47**(10): 2015–2028.

6. https://www.bnl.gov/newsroom/news.php?a=1496

7. http://www.alzfdn.org/AboutAlzheimers/lifeexpectancy.html

8. http://www.sciencedirect.com/science/article/pii/S1474442204007677

9. Borenstein AR, Copenhaver CI, Mortimer JA. (2006) Early-life risk factors for Alzheimer disease. *Alzheimer Dis Assoc Disord* **20**(1): 63–72.

4

What is Dementia?

"The real truth is that science is not man's nature, it is mere knowledge and training. By knowing the laws of the material universe you do not change your deeper humanity. You can borrow knowledge from others, but you cannot borrow temperament."

— *Nationalism* by Rabindranath Tagore, Nobel Laureate (Literature, 1913)

Dementia can be dissected into the prefix *de-*, which means "to depart" and *-mens,* which stands for mind. Literally, dementia means "to depart from one's mind."[1] It is a general term to describe a wide range of symptoms that lead to overall mental decline that is severe enough to interfere with everyday life.

Dementia is a term that has become ubiquitously associated with Alzheimer's disease, but despite the colloquial intermingling of the two concepts, they are disparate entities. The difference can be understood with the following analogy. Imagine a car that is broken down on the side of the road. There are many different things that could have caused the car to break. The engine could have malfunctioned, the transmission could have been rendered non-operational, or it simply could have run out of gas. Well, dementia is analogous to the broken car — it is a clinical term that describes a constellation of symptoms, but there is no explanation of the etiology inherent in the term itself. The reason why dementia and Alzheimer's disease are thought of as equivalent is because 70–80% of dementia cases are caused by Alzheimer's disease.[2]

For example, if an individual has memory loss, personality changes, or cognitive dysfunction, he or she may be given the diagnosis of dementia. However, the cause of the dementia has to be determined following the diagnosis. Some important features to take into consideration are what part of the brain is affected, whether the dementia worsens over time, or if it is reversible. The most common cause of dementia is Alzheimer's disease; however, there are many other causes, just like there are many reasons that a car may break down.

In addition to Alzheimer's disease, there are many other primary classifications of dementia. These disorders directly lead to dementia, unlike "secondary" disorders, which are only associated with dementia. One primary cause of dementia includes vascular dementia, which is due to many "micro" strokes within the brain due to cerebrovascular (blood vessels of the brain) disease. Another primary cause of dementia is late-stage Parkinson's disease (PD), which is a movement disorder that is caused by the deterioration of a specific group of dopamine-producing neurons in the brain. Additionally, frontotemporal dementia (FTD) is a primary cause of dementia that is related to Alzheimer's disease, but attacks the frontal lobes first instead of the hippocampus. Furthermore, dementia with Lewy Bodies (DLB) is a combination of PD and Alzheimer's disease that can often be misdiagnosed. The list of primary causes of dementia continues with a condition that we will elaborate on in later chapters known as chronic traumatic encephalopathy (CTE). CTE is also known as punch-drunk syndrome and can occur in football players and boxers. In fact, it is what the famous boxer Muhammad Ali was diagnosed with. These primary causes of dementia are not reversible and worsen over time.

There is also a secondary classification of disorders that are linked to dementia. These include Huntington's disease, PD, normal pressure hydrocephalus (NPH), and traumatic brain injury (TBI). NPH usually occurs in individuals over the age of 60 and after a head injury (i.e. TBI). In NPH, cerebrospinal fluid (CSF) drainage is somehow impeded and the excess fluid builds up and slowly puts pressure on the brain. The parts of the brain that are most often affected in NPH are those that control the legs, the bladder, and the "cognitive" mental processes such as memory, reasoning, problem solving, and speaking. Thus, patients are often misdiagnosed as having PD or Alzheimer's disease. However, unlike Alzheimer's disease, NPH is treatable.[3]

The prevalence of dementia pugilistica, or CTE, a neurodegenerative disease that exhibits features of dementia that may affect boxers (*pugil* comes from the Latin root for "boxer"), wrestlers, or other athletes who may suffer concussions, suggests an association between TBI and dementia.

Research performed at the Cleveland Clinic and at the University of Rochester shows changes occur in athletes' magnetic resonance imaging scans who have been diagnosed with CTE. Studies from the Cleveland Clinic demonstrated a relationship between mild TBI, such as a mild concussion, and the leakage of a substance known as S100B in the patient's blood. The leakage is thought to occur due to the opening or weakening of the blood–brain barrier, which is meant to isolate the delicate cells within the brain from the harsh and toxic substances carried in the bloodstream.[4] Although we need more conclusive studies on this association, it suggests a possible relationship with Alzheimer's disease, since S100B antibodies, which are immunological proteins that can specifically bind to S100B, have also been identified in Alzheimer's patients.

TBI is a common problem in adolescents and young adults, but notably is bimodally distributed, with another incidence peak in adults over the age of 65 (Fig. 4.1).[5] Interestingly enough, dementia has been shown to be a risk factor for actually experiencing TBI. Conversely, having a history of TBI is also an important risk factor in the development of dementia.[6] Normally, TBI in the elderly is caused by car accidents and falls, with the presence of dementia being an important risk factor for both causes. Unfortunately, there are a variety of debilitating cognitive consequences that follow TBI that can even outlast the physical impairments that arise immediately following TBI. These changes in cognition can include, but are not limited to, changes in attention, memory, and executive functioning, which includes our ability to plan or problem solve.

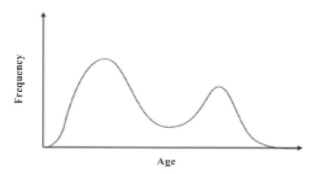

Fig. 4.1. An example of a bimodal distribution. Traumatic brain injury (TBI) is bimodally distributed in young and elderly individuals. (Modified from Ref. 7.)

The reason that we are discussing TBI is that meta-analyses of large numbers of studies have suggested that TBI is a risk factor for the eventual development of Alzheimer's disease.[8,9] The association between Alzheimer's disease and TBI has been consistently reported in the literature, with one prospective study that followed a large group of individuals reporting a relative risk of 4.1 for developing Alzheimer's disease in patients with past medical histories of TBI. This means that individuals who have had a TBI in the past are approximately four-times more likely to develop Alzheimer's disease.

The mechanism by which TBI may lead to Alzheimer's disease is multifaceted and not completely understood. One of the potential mechanisms relating the two has been published in the literature. A study conducted in 2003 showed that TBI can modulate hippocampal synaptic plasticity and lead to amyloid precursor protein (APP) accumulation in damaged axons.[10] As discussed earlier, APP leads to the hallmark plaques that are found in Alzheimer's disease. These plaques disrupt communication between neurons within the brain at the level of the synapse. Additionally, severe TBI has been shown to lead to the accumulation of the β-amyloid protein within the CSF in humans.[11] CSF is the fluid that bathes and nourishes the brain, and it is normally tightly regulated. However, when β-amyloid accumulates in humans, it has been shown to cause destruction and atrophy (shrinkage due to cell death) of the hippocampus, which, as mentioned previously, is the structure within the brain that is responsible for memory formation.

In addition, the presence of β-amyloid in the CSF can make the glial cells in the brain more sensitive and reactive. In studies conducted on mice, the presence of β-amyloid in the CSF was shown to lead to inflammatory responses within the brain that resulted in a wide cascade of negative effects. A general rule of thumb is that prolonged inflammation is actually damaging to the body and can lead to a plethora of deleterious consequences for the human body. Thus, TBI-related inflammation within the brain may predispose neurons to damage and could predispose individuals to Alzheimer's disease; however, the degree of correlation is unclear. TBI may decrease cognitive reserve or lead to Alzheimer's-like cognitive impairments that mimic Alzheimer's disease.[12]

In fact, one form of TBI, known as a chronic subdural hematoma (cSDH), has been described as "the great neurological imitator" because it often presents itself as a constellation of symptoms that can resemble a psychiatric disorder, dementia, a migraine, epilepsy, PD, or stroke. A cSDH is a collection of blood within the meninges (the protective layers of tissue that cover the brain). Classically called "pseudodementia," cSDH is an important cause of reversible dementia in the elderly.[13] Left untreated, cSDH can often be confused with Alzheimer's disease due to the similarity in signs and symptoms between the two conditions. Thus, when a patient presents to a doctor with symptoms that might resemble dementia, other medical conditions that may mimic dementia, such as cSDH, must be ruled out. Nonetheless, injuries to the brain can put individuals at higher risk for the development of dementia.

To add to this convoluted list of causes that can lead to dementia, some patients suffer from idiopathic dementia, which means that we do not know what is causing it. Each of these causes represents a distinct pathological process that can lead to the constellation of symptoms that represents dementia. Many individuals who suffer from dementia do not have a very clear-cut etiology. On autopsy, there are usually several underlying factors, which are often complicated by cerebrovascular disease, which ultimately led to that patient's untimely death.

What Causes Dementia and Alzheimer's Disease?

The cause of Alzheimer's disease is still not fully elucidated. Although we can clearly see what the consequences of the disease are, the actual cause of the disease is still unknown. There are many theories that seek to explain the cause, but ultimately, damage to cells (neurons and glial cells) in the brain results in dementia.[14] Some theories for what causes the cellular damage include misfolding of certain proteins, dysfunctional clearance of damaged proteins from the brain, or even dysfunctional levels of neurotransmitters (particularly acetylcholine) in the brain.[15–17]

Regardless of the cause, cellular damage leads to dysfunctional communication amongst the neurons within the brain. This leads to changes in thoughts, emotions, memory, and more depending on the location of damage (since different parts of the brain are responsible for different things). In Alzheimer's disease, for example, the earliest site of cellular damage and dysfunction occurs in the hippocampus — this is the region that is responsible for the formation of new memories. When cells within the hippocampus are damaged, the ability of those cells to carry out their normal function is impaired. Since those cells normally function in the creation and consolidation of new memories, damage results in memory impairments in patients in the early stages of Alzheimer's disease. As the disease spreads throughout the brain, other brain regions become affected, resulting in the outward clinical symptoms that are seen in Alzheimer's patients in later stages of the disease. These "later" symptoms include an inability to communicate and make plans, changes in emotions and mood, and eventually a diminished cough reflex that can lead to aspiration (inhaling fluid) and pneumonia.

Although most causes of dementia are permanent and lead to steadily worsening clinical symptomatology in patients, some causes of dementia are actually reversible when treated. These treatable causes of memory impairment (Table 4.1) include depression, neurosurgical conditions such as NPH or subdural hematomas, inflammation or infection of the brain, alcoholism, metabolic disorders such as hypo- or hyperthyroidism, vitamin deficiency (B1, B6, B12, and folate), and more.[18]

The treatable dementias are generally screened for by neurologists prior to making a diagnosis of Alzheimer's disease or another type of dementia. Although Alzheimer's disease is the most common cause of dementia (80%–90), followed by vascular causes of dementia (approximately 20%), potentially reversible causes of dementia make up anywhere from 9% to 23% of cases.[19] The reversible causes of dementia are varied and theoretically treatable if detected and addressed in a timely fashion. NPH, for example, can cause expansion of the lateral ventricles (LV) (CSF-filled cavities within the two hemispheres in the brain) and can lead to alterations in the normal function of white matter tracts (the cellular projections, or axons, of neurons), resulting in disruptions of memory and cognition that resemble dementia. This condition can be treated surgically with the placement of a shunt that drains excess fluid from the ventricles into another part of the body. Similarly, brain tumors,

Table 4.1.   **Treatable Causes of Memory Impairment**

Neurosurgical problems	**Brain infections and inflammation**	**Metabolic disorders**	**Other**
Normal pressure hydrocephalus	Inflammation of the brain (encephalitis) or meninges (meningitis)	Hypo- or hyper-thyroidism or parathyroidism	Depression
Brain tumors	Neurosyphilis	High calcium (hypercalcemia)	Drugs/alcohol/toxins
Brain abscess	AIDS-related dementia	Vitamin B1, B6, B12, or folate deficiency	Epilepsy
Brain bleed (subdural hematoma)	—	Liver or renal failure	Sleep apnea

abscesses, or bleeds can all cause increases in pressure within the brain and alter normal brain function. The removal of these offenders can alleviate the stresses placed on the brain and result in a return to normal cognitive function.

Infections and inflammation within the brain or its coverings (meninges) can also lead to disturbances in the normal function of the cells within the brain. This altered cellular function can also disrupt the cellular processes involved in normal cellular communication and homeostasis and result in the presence of cognitive alterations that could resemble dementia. The same mechanism underlies how metabolic disorders can lead to dementia-like symptoms in that there is a change in the normally tightly controlled homeostatic mechanisms that allow the delicate neurons in the brain to function properly. Depression, drugs, and alcohol can also lead to decreased cognitive abilities such as memory formation — this can sometimes trick medical professionals into thinking that the patient has Alzheimer's disease when in fact they have a different medical condition underlying their apparent dementia. The widespread use of depression and alcoholism screening questionnaires in individuals who are at risk of the development of Alzheimer's disease helps medical providers pick up potentially treatable causes of dementia in order to address the clinical symptoms that a patient may have. In addition, laboratory tests can help screen patients for metabolic disorders such as vitamin deficiencies, which could be addressed via vitamin B12 shots or oral dietary supplements.

However, if other causes of dementia are ruled out and neuropsychological and neurological examinations suggest a dementia of the Alzheimer's type, then the likelihood of the dementia being reversed by treatment becomes unlikely. Alzheimer's disease, as mentioned previously, has a ubiquitous and unclear etiology (cause). One of the potential ways in which the cellular damage underlying Alzheimer's disease occurs is due to the misfolding and altered functioning of certain proteins. Proteins are critical components of all cells. The blueprint for what proteins are produced by each cell in the body is determined by the genetic make up of an individual. The DNA found within the nucleus of each cell determines what specific proteins that cell will make. Certain proteins are only made by certain cells in the body, and this regulation is tightly controlled. This is also why there are different "types" of cells within the body, and why a hair cell differs from a brain or heart cell. The DNA is the blueprint, and the blueprint is then used in order to make a molecule known as messenger RNA (mRNA). This mRNA is a unique molecule that reflects the genetic code from which it is derived from. The mRNA is then used as a template in order to encode a unique sequence of amino acids, which results in a completed protein. Proteins have a wide variety of functions within the cell and are essential to normal function. They help with cellular signaling and cellular repair and defense, and they help to provide structure to the cell, along with many more important functions. When proteins are damaged or not properly formed (as in the case of a genetic mutation resulting in a protein with altered functionality), the protein is sometimes rendered useless and can even lead to cellular damage if not destroyed and disposed of properly.

Many neurodegenerative diseases have some component of abnormal protein accumulation, which such proteins are referred to as neurodegenerative-related proteins. These can include alpha-synuclein in PD, APP in Alzheimer's disease, and prion protein in prion-related diseases such as Creutzfeldt–Jakob or mad cow disease.[20] These proteins are similar in that they usually are found in the membrane of the cell and are thus known as integral or membrane-associated proteins. These proteins reach the cell membrane only after they are created within a specialized region of the cell known as the endoplasmic reticulum (ER).

In order for a protein to leave the ER and be properly inserted into the cell membrane, it must be completely functional and be free of damage. One way in which a protein can lose its function is by the improper folding of the amino acid sequence that makes up the complete protein. The improper folding alters the three-dimensional structure of a protein, and can thus alter its function. Some proteins inevitably become damaged and dysfunctional due to protein misfolding, even in normal and healthy cells. These misfolded proteins are usually destroyed and removed from the cell in order for normal proteins to take their place. The misfolded proteins are destroyed by being shuttled to a lysosome or proteasome (cellular structures that destroy proteins), and then degraded via a mechanism known as autophagy (*auto* means self and *phagy* means to eat).

When this process is disrupted, it can lead to increased cellular stress and something known as the unfolded protein response (UPR). The UPR aims to restore normal cellular function by stopping protein formation, destroying misfolded proteins, and producing molecules that assist in protein folding. If these aims do not properly restore cellular function, the cell can undergo apoptosis (controlled cell death). Understanding and modulating the UPR via drugs is actually one of the many avenues that are being considered and pursued in the treatment of Alzheimer's disease and other neurodegenerative disorders.

Recently, neuroscientists at Columbia University Medical Center (CUMC) and New York State Psychiatric Institute (NYSPI) found that improving a "brain's garbage disposal system" may slow down Alzheimer's.[21] The main actors in this cerebral garbage disposal system are proteasomes, which are molecules that break down old proteins so that they can be recycled into new ones. This happens in what we call the ubiquitination proteasome system (UPS), a two-step system in which old proteins are ubiquitinated (tagged through an enzymatic process) and proteasomes (proteins that break down other proteins) digest only those ubiquitinated proteins (Fig.4.2).[22] The neuroscientists at CUMC and NYSPI found a drug — rolipram — that could reactivate proteasomes and slow down Alzheimer's disease. This leads us to consider another factor for Alzheimer's disease: impaired proteasomes restrict them from digesting old, possibly toxic proteins.

One study suggests just this — that while the Alzheimer's brain may not have difficulty recognizing dangerous proteins (the ubiquitination step), the proteasome may be unable to function properly in digesting those proteins (the digesting step). It appears that once the older proteins

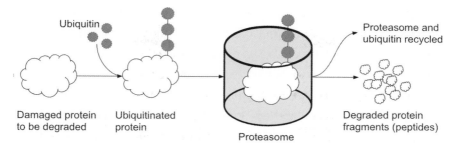

Fig. 4.2.   Proteins that need to be degraded are "tagged" by a molecule known as ubiquitin, which allows these proteins to be degraded by a proteasome. (Modified from Ref. 22.)

are ubiquitinated, something in the UPS goes awry. Scientists have hypothesized that this happens in one of two ways: either the proteasome becomes overactive and destroys healthy proteins, or its activity is restricted and there is a build-up of toxic proteins.[23] The study on rolipram suggests that the latter is happening, although the mechanism underlying this is unknown. In this model, as toxic aggregates accumulate over time, there is even more proteasome impairment, analogous to the dangerous snowball effects of Alzheimer's disease neurodegeneration. By activating proteasomes and making the UPS functional, neurotoxicity can perhaps be avoided.

In February of 2015, a study conducted by a large group of researchers from the University of Cambridge, the Karolinska Institute in Stockholm, Lund University, the Swedish University of Agricultural Sciences, and Tallinn University discovered a small molecule known as Brichos, which can block the progression of Alzheimer's disease. This is an interesting finding, as it may have potential implications for decreasing plaque formation in the brains of individuals with Alzheimer's disease. However, these results are still in their preliminary stages, and it will take many more years before human studies may be considered. Nonetheless, the discovery of the Brichos molecule is very promising.

The Brichos molecule functions by adhering to the dysfunctional and damaging β-amyloid proteins that are readily found in the brains of patients with Alzheimer's disease. Brichos prevents threads of β-amyloid from accumulating and prevents a critical step in the formation of the harmful neuritic plaques found in Alzheimer's brains. It acts as a "molecular chaperone," ensuring that the β-amyloid does not form fibrils that eventually accumulate and form plaques. In one particular study conducted on mice, the researchers exposed the brain cells of the mice to β-amyloid, leading to the formation of the toxic and misfolded amyloid plaques. When the researchers added the Brichos molecule, the amyloid fibrils still formed; however, there were no signs of toxicity within the brain tissue. This finding suggests that the molecule suppressed the "chain reaction" that occurs when β-amyloid proteins accumulate and contribute to Alzheimer's disease.[24,25]

Despite the many theories that have been proposed and thoroughly studied, the exact cause of Alzheimer's disease has yet to be elucidated. The lack of a complete understanding of why Alzheimer's disease develops partially explains why the efforts to control it have been so easily thwarted. Regardless, as more research is being done in order to better understand Alzheimer's disease, the answers may be closer than we once thought.

References

1. http://www1.appstate.edu/~hillrw/Alzheimers/dementia%20site/Templates/Index.htm
2. http://www.alz.org/downloads/Facts_Figures_2014.pdf
3. Mysiw WJ, Jackson RD. (1990) Relationship of new-onset systemic hypertension and normal pressure hydrocephalus. *Brain Injury* 4(3): 233–238.
4. Pham N, Fazio V, Cucullo L, *et al.* (2010) Extracranial sources of S100B do not affect serum levels. *PLoS ONE* 5(9): e12691.
5. Adhiyaman V, Asghar M, Ganeshram KN, Bhowmick BK. (2002) Chronic subdural haematoma in the elderly. *Postgrad Med J* **78**(916): 71–75.
6. Inao S, Kawai T, Kabeya R, *et al.* (2001) Relation between brain displacement and local cerebral blood flow in patients with chronic subdural haematoma. *J Neurol Neurosurg Psychiatry* **71**(6): 741–746.
7. https://commons.wikimedia.org/wiki/File:Bimodal_geological.PNG
8. Lye TC, Shores EA. (2000) Traumatic brain injury as a risk factor for Alzheimer's disease: A review. *Neuropsychol Rev* **10**: 115–129.

9. Fleminger S, Oliver DL, Lovestone S, *et al.* (2003) Head injury as a risk factor for Alzheimer's disease: The evidence 10 years on; a partial replication. *J Neurol Neurosurg Psychiatry* **74**: 857–862.

10. Fleminger S, Oliver DL, Lovestone S, *et al.* (2003) Head injury as a risk factor for Alzheimer's disease: the evidence 10 years on; a partial replication. *J Neurol Neurosurg Psychiatry* **74**(7): 857–862.

11. Emmerling MR, Morganti-Kossmann MC, Kossmann T, *et al.* (2000) Traumatic brain injury elevates the Alzheimer's amyloid peptide A beta 42 in human CSF. A possible role for nerve cell injury. *Ann N Y Acad Sci* **903**: 118–122.

12. Stone JR, Okonkwo DO, Singleton RH, *et al.* (2002) Caspase-3-mediated cleavage of amyloid precursor protein and formation of amyloid beta peptide in traumatic axonal injury. *J Neurotrauma* **19**: 601–614.

13. https://commons.wikimedia.org/wiki/File:Systemic_Inflammation_AD_01.jpg

14. Inao S, Kawai T, Kabeya R, *et al.* (2001) Relation between brain displacement and local cerebral blood flow in patients with chronic subdural haematoma. *J Neurol Neurosurg Psychiatry* **71**(6): 741–746.

15. http://www.alz.org/what-is-dementia.asp#causes

16. http://www.dementiaguide.com/aboutdementia/alzheimers/cholinergic_theory/

17. http://newsroom.cumc.columbia.edu/blog/2015/12/21/improving-brains-garbage-disposal-may-slow-alzheimers-disease/

18. Lipatova Z, Shah AH, Kim JJ, *et al.* (2013) Regulation of ER-phagy by a Ypt/Rab GTPase module. *Mol Biol Cell* **24**(19): 3133–3144.

19. Tripathi M, Vibha D. (2009) Reversible dementias. *Indian J Psychiatry* **51**(Suppl. 1): S52.

20. Shankle WR, Romney AK, Hara J, *et al.* (2005) Methods to improve the detection of mild cognitive impairment. *Proc Natl Acad Sci USA* **102**(13): 4919–4924.

21. http://www.ninds.nih.gov/disorders/cjd/detail_cjd.htm

22. http://newsroom.cumc.columbia.edu/blog/2015/12/21/improving-brains-garbage-disposal-may-slow-alzheimers-disease/

23. http://www.nature.com/ncomms/2014/141208/ncomms6659/fig_tab/ncomms6659_F1.html

24. bio1151.nicerweb.com

25. Deger JM, Gerson JE, Kayed R. (2015) The interrelationship of proteasome impairment and oligomeric intermediates in neurodegeneration. *Aging Cell* **14**(5): 715–724.

26. http://www.cam.ac.uk/research/news/molecular-inhibitor-breaks-cycle-that-leads-to-alzheimers

27. Cohen SI, Arosio P, Presto J, *et al.* (2015) A molecular chaperone breaks the catalytic cycle that generates toxic Aβ oligomers. *Nat Struct Mol Biol* **22**(3): 207–213.

5 Introduction to Alzheimer's Disease

"If you can dream — and not make dreams your master;
If you can think — and not make thoughts your aim;
If you can meet with Triumph and Disaster
And treat those two impostors just the same;"

— Excerpt from *If* by Rudyard Kipling, Nobel Laureate
(Literature, 1907)

Alzheimer's disease has begun to attract the attention of national leaders around the world. As a disease that primarily affects elderly adults, it is growing in importance as the world's population ages. In fact, as life expectancy increases on a yearly basis and as baby boomers begin entering their sixth decade of life, Alzheimer's disease has evolved into a public health crisis. Alzheimer's has acquired national attention in recent years, and has been acted upon by President Barack Obama, who in 2011 signed into existence the National Alzheimer's Project Act, or NAPA for short. This piece of legislation established a national strategic plan focused on containing the growing issue of Alzheimer's disease. It sought to increase funding to researchers focused on treatments for Alzheimer's disease, as well as increasing funding and resources to Alzheimer's disease national organizations and the families of patients afflicted by the disease.

In order to successfully end the devastation that Alzheimer's disease causes, a variety of approaches to its early diagnosis, treatment, and prevention must be taken. In order to incentivize the best scientists in the country to focus on the various aspects of Alzheimer's disease, there need to be substantive and long-standing federal resources in the forms of grants and funding opportunities in order to bolster the formation and propagation of research laboratories that are focused on Alzheimer's disease. In 2015, Alzheimer's and other dementias cost the USA $226 billion annually; it is projected that by 2015, this financial burden will skyrocket to $1.1 trillion, more than quadrupling the annual burden.[1]

Saying that this problem is serious is an understatement, and these financial costs are objective measures of the damage that dementia inflicts on the USA. Subjective measures of the damaging effects of dementia and Alzheimer's disease are difficult to quantify, ranging from the devastation it creates within families to the medical burden it will create as patients put pressure on the medical system and its limited resources. Despite the enormous financial and sociological impact that dementia and Alzheimer's disease has in the USA, only $480 million a year is devoted to the study of Alzheimer's disease by the National Institutes of Health (NIH).[2] Although $480 million a year seems like a lot of money, it is less than 0.002% of the financial burden of dementia and Alzheimer's disease in 2015. In comparison, America's gross national product (GNP) is $17 trillion.

Awareness of Alzheimer's disease and the actions that could alleviate its effects at the national level are critical in order to better understand the disease and find a cure. Recently, however, the poor economic climate in the USA has forced many researchers to abandon their quest for discovering cures due to a lack of government funds to keep their laboratories afloat. There is also less of an incentive for new researchers to focus their laboratories on Alzheimer's disease due to the lack of national financial support and an increasingly competitive landscape where less than 10% of grant applications are funded. Researchers may have better luck obtaining funding if they focus on other diseases such as cancer, heart disease, or HIV/AIDS, which receive $6 billion, $4 billion, and $4 billion a year, respectively. Alzheimer's disease, on the other hand, as mentioned above, only receives $480 million a year from the federal government. Despite this measly fiscal climate, due to the advancement

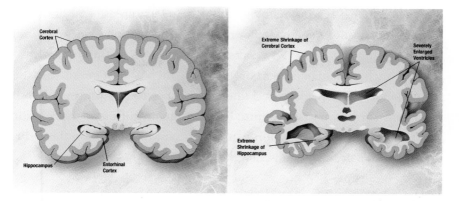

Fig. 5.1. A normal (left) and Alzheimer's brain (right). (Figure credit: Ref. 3.)

of new technologies, such as radioactive isotope imaging or stem cell-based therapeutics, a new sense of hope has revitalized many scientists look for Alzheimer's disease treatments.

One approach to the treatment of Alzheimer's disease that has been gaining traction has been focused on thinking "outside the box" and trying to figure out completely new and novel ideas for potentially attacking the disease process. The classical school of thought that has predominated for many years with regards to the treatment of Alzheimer's disease has been premised on attempting to reduce or eliminate the abnormal protein aggregates that are the hallmark pathological features of Alzheimer's disease (Fig. 5.1). However, the role of these aggregates (plaques and tangles) has become increasingly uncertain as more is understood about the disease process. The accumulation of β-amyloid into plaques within the brain is classically associated with Alzheimer's disease, as is the formation of tangles within neurons. Most research and therapeutic efforts have attempted to reduce the plaque and tangle load within the brain. Recently, however, new approaches have shown promise. Instead of focusing on the plaques and tangles, focusing on harnessing the brain's endogenous regenerative capacity or improving the brain's ability to filter toxins have shown promise in terms of alleviating the clinical symptomatology of Alzheimer's disease. Additionally, it is becoming increasingly apparent that the formation of plaques and tangles within the brain represents the later stages in the disease process. As such, it may be important to tackle the problem underlying the formation of these plaques and tangles long before the presentation of any clinical symptoms in patients. There are many different therapeutic strategies that are being explored at the present moment, and these different approaches will be discussed in future chapters.

Clinical Symptoms

The early stages of Alzheimer's disease are classically associated with lapses in memory. As individuals age, it is completely normal for minor memory lapses to occur; for example, forgetting where you placed your keys, or the name of a new friend. However, the memory changes that are indicative of Alzheimer's disease are much more dramatic, are not transient and progressively worsen over time. Examples of Alzheimer's-type memory loss include forgetting conversations that just took place, forgetting the names of family members or close friends, misplacing items frequently, or altering the order of items (such as putting on underwear over jeans or socks on top of shoes).

However, memory problems are only a minor part of the constellation of clinical symptoms that constitute Alzheimer's disease. Some other frequently seen symptoms include a deterioration in spatial awareness (the sense of position in space), such as getting lost in familiar places, or misinterpreting spatial relationships — making it difficult to drive or navigate in normal environments or roads. In addition to the memory changes, disorientation, and loss of spatial awareness, patients suffer from language disturbances, making it difficult to communicate effectively. Many patients experience "tip-of-the-tongue" phenomena in which they cannot find the right word even though they know what they are trying to verbalize. This often leads to a sense of frustration and agitation, and some patients even deny that they are having any problems with communication or memory impairments. Table 5.1 lists out some of the symptoms that are usually seen in Alzheimer's disease

Table 5.1.   Common Alzheimer's Symptoms
Memory loss and confusion
Difficulty recognizing loved ones
Difficulty learning new tasks
Difficulty completing multifaceted tasks
Difficulty adjusting to new environments and events
Delusions, paranoia, and hallucinations
Impulsivity

One group of important cognitive functions that is commonly tested during the standard array of neuropsychiatric diagnostic tests is higher cognitive processes, such as reasoning, decision making, and the planning and execution of movements. These cognitive processes are all adversely affected by the underlying pathological processes of Alzheimer's disease, and unfortunately, they eventually lead to severe social problems between the patient and his or her closest friends and family members.

In the middle to late stages of Alzheimer's disease, the problems associated with memory loss, cognitive deterioration, and social ineptitude eventually give way to personality changes and even behavioral changes such as depression, anxiety, and delusions. Fortunately, some patients who are initially diagnosed with Alzheimer's disease are able to enjoy a relatively normal cognitive status for many months to years after they are diagnosed. Additionally, there is a wide spectrum of cognitive deterioration in patients with Alzheimer's disease, with some patients surviving from 5 to 20 years after the initial diagnosis.[4] This, of course, depends on many factors, including at what point in the disease process the diagnosis was made, the amount of cognitive reserve, the initiation of a proper treatment regimen, and more. However, as the disease progresses, the very essence of that individual's mind deteriorates and unfortunately gives way to the unrelenting pathological processes of Alzheimer's disease.

One interesting feature of Alzheimer's disease that makes it extremely elusive is the gradual progression of symptoms and the very gradual decline of function in patients. Unlike other disorders, which appear quickly and have symptoms that are readily manifested in patients, the symptoms of Alzheimer's disease start out very mildly and progress slowly. This makes it extremely difficult for family members and those who are close to the patient to notice the deterioration until the disease is extremely far progressed. To exemplify this, imagine an individual who is extremely highly functioning and independent. This individual is capable of driving, grocery shopping, exercising, and doing other normal everyday tasks. If that individual suddenly, within the course of several hours or days, becomes unable to drive, cannot dress himself or herself and forgets where he or she is, it would be readily apparent that something is wrong. This would likely prompt the patient and his or her family to go and see a physician or go to an emergency room, and a thorough work-up would ensue. Thus, it is easy to realize that something is wrong when a patient experiences a sudden decline in function over a period of hours or days.

However, if the decline in function occurred over the course of 2–3 years, it would be extremely difficult to tease out whether the patient is simply deciding to no longer participate in normal everyday activities by choice or if they are cognitively and physically incapable of doing so. This makes it difficult to realize that there is something wrong, delaying the initial visit to a physician or the sense of urgency in making a diagnosis and initiating treatment. Additionally, it is important that when the patient does see a physician, the correct diagnosis is made, as there are many other causes of dementia. Anytime that a patient sees a physician for the evaluation of a medical condition, the physician creates a mental list of the possible causes of the problem. This is known as a differential diagnosis. It is similar to what you would see if you went onto WebMD.com and selected a specific set of symptoms. The website would generate a list of possible medical conditions that could be the cause of the problem, and that list is known as a differential diagnosis. However, unlike a website, a physician must take into account every aspect of that patient's life, medical history, laboratory evaluations, and more in order to make a correct diagnosis.

Unfortunately, there is no definitive test for Alzheimer's disease. Instead, doctors call it a "clinical diagnosis," meaning that it is a diagnosis that requires multiple tests, a physical examination and a medical history for its determination. This can sometimes be frustrating to patients, since they have to undergo a battery of tests and sometimes wait many months in order to obtain a diagnosis. Additionally, the clinical diagnosis of Alzheimer's disease is actually more accurately labeled as "probable Alzheimer's disease," because the only way to definitely diagnose Alzheimer's disease is upon autopsy after death (or, in very rare cases, a brain biopsy is done while the patient is still alive). There is no specific test or laboratory value that allows doctors to make a diagnosis of Alzheimer's disease. In some cases, the diagnosis is not clearly known and is given as a "catch net" diagnosis when all other diseases have been ruled out.

Differential Diagnosis

Because of the ambiguity of diagnosis, there are many diseases that can mimic Alzheimer's, both in its clinical presentation and also in its radiographic findings, such as computed tomography (CT) and magnetic resonance imaging (MRI) scans of the brain. One of the major imitators of Alzheimer's disease is depression. In fact, 30–50% of patients with Alzheimer's disease also suffer from depression.[5] Those with depression often suffer from impairment in memory and even motor function (movement). Depressed patients may even be incorrectly diagnosed with Alzheimer's disease due to the negative effects of depression on tests that assess memory. Clinically differentiating between Alzheimer's disease and depression is rather difficult, but can be done by administering a variety of screening and confirmatory tests in order to assess levels

Table 5.2.   Criteria Used to Diagnose Depression in Alzheimer's Disease[5]

A. Three or more of the following criteria over a 2-week period and differing from normal functioning. Additionally, at least one of the symptoms needs to be: (1) depressed mood or (2) a decrease in pleasure or positive mood

- Significantly depressed mood
- Less pleasure in social or normal activities
- Social isolation
- Appetite changes
- Sleep changes
- Movement or psychological changes
- Irritability
- Fatigue or lack of energy
- Feelings of worthlessness, hopelessness, or extreme guilt
- Frequent thoughts of death or suicide

B. Criteria are met for Alzheimer's disease

C. Symptoms are causing changes in normal functioning

D. Symptoms do not coincide with delirium

E. Symptoms are not due to medications or drugs

F. Symptoms are not accounted for by other psychiatric disorders

of depression. Tests include the Hamilton Scale for Depression and the Geriatric Depression Scale (GDS), which is specific to the elderly population. Nevertheless, patients may be suffering from both Alzheimer's and depression independently. As a result, the National Institute of Mental Health (NIMH) has developed a specific set of criteria for diagnosing depression in Alzheimer's. The criteria are illustrated in Table 5.2. As outlined in the table, patients who have Alzheimer's disease and also have depression usually exhibit unique qualities and changes in motivation. Although the symptoms vary, the most common findings are fatigue or psychomotor retardation, which are defined by a physical slowing and reduction of movements. Elderly patients that have depression while also having Alzheimer's disease also behave differently and exhibit mood changes more often than normal. These mood disturbances mainly revolve around increased anxiety and depression, as well as disruption in sleep and appetite patterns.

Because memory loss is often the hallmark of Alzheimer's disease, many normal elderly adults are often worried that they are suffering from the disease. As previously discussed, as we age, it is typical to experience a progressively mild decline in memory. Common complaints include forgetting the location of keys, appointments, and sometimes entering a room only to forget why they entered. The difference between these experiences and those when suffering from dementia is blurred initially, but becomes more distinct as the disease progresses. Dementia can interrupt hobbies, work, and social interactions with loved ones. Herein lies the biggest difference between Alzheimer's and normal age-related memory loss. In normal memory loss, one's life is not drastically impacted, instead being only as a minor inconvenience. Only when the memory loss affects one's ability to function does it become concerning regarding signs of early dementia.

The second most common cause of dementia following Alzheimer's disease is vascular dementia. In vascular dementia, the arteries that direct blood to the brain are damaged, usually by plaque build-up called atherosclerosis or stroke. This damage encumbers the ability of the brain to receive vital oxygen and nutrients, resulting in injury to the brain. Because of this, MRI scans of the brain can shed light on the diagnosis and identify which part of the brain has been affected. The clinical symptoms differ from Alzheimer's in terms of the rate of progression. In Alzheimer's, cognitive and memory declines occur gradually. In vascular dementia, there is an inciting event such as a stroke, which causes a rapid decline. Additionally, there are usually focal physical deficits, such as not being able to move one side of the body, which accompany the decline in cognitive function.

With memory loss being the key feature of Alzheimer's, other types of dementia must be ruled out before coming to an accurate diagnosis. Of the most common dementias — Lewy bodies disease — must be considered. Lewy bodies disease, otherwise known as dementia with Lewy bodies (DLB), accounts for 1 in 25 cases of dementia.[6] Patients with DLB have what are known as Lewy bodies in their brains. These Lewy bodies are composed of a protein known as α-synuclein and can result in the degeneration of the neurons that are involved in Parkinson's disease (PD). Therefore, the clinical presentation of DLB exhibits a progressive decline in cognitive function, in addition to mild to moderate movement abnormalities (similar to those in PD). Another interesting symptom in DLB patients is the presence of recurrent visual hallucinations.[7] Additionally, DLB patients have variations in cognitive function in which attention and alertness fluctuate, which are also seen in Alzheimer's disease. However, Alzheimer's disease has a characteristic "sundowning" effect, in which these changes occur in the evening. In DLB, these can occur for longer periods of time and may include episodes of staring off in space for an extended period of time. However, the characteristic findings of DLB patients are Parkinsonian-like motor features, including tremors, which are not usually seen until the later stages of Alzheimer's.

Furthermore, nutritional causes of dementia must also be considered in the differential diagnosis of Alzheimer's disease. Most notably, a deficiency in vitamin B12 can present with symptoms that are similar to Alzheimer's disease.[8] The overlapping symptomatology is memory loss, agitation, and even changes in behavior. Vitamin B12 deficiency is different in that the symptoms include changes in sensory function, which may be absent in Alzheimer's disease. These motor changes can include poor balance, weakness, tingling, or numbness in the peripheral extremities. A diagnosis of vitamin B12 deficiency is generally better news, since it is a reversible cause of dementia and can easily be treatment by taking oral doses of vitamin B12. Due to the simplicity of the screening test for vitamin B12 deficiency and its benefit in terms of diagnosis, all patients presenting with any form of dementia should be screened for this vitamin deficiency.

Because Alzheimer's disease is a clinical diagnosis as previously described, diagnostic and imaging tests must be conducted in order to rule out other potential causes of the symptoms. Treating and diagnosing

Alzheimer's disease requires doctors with different medical specialties to work together as a team. Typically, patients present to their primary care physician with symptoms of dementia. These physicians are trained in how to treat and diagnose Alzheimer's disease and may decide to treat the patient themselves or refer the patient to a specialist, depending on a multitude of factors. The medical specialist who commonly receives the most training on Alzheimer's disease is the neurologist. Neurologists usually spend 4 or more years after medical school training in how to treat all diseases of the brain, ranging from stroke to Alzheimer's. In addition, some neurologists choose to undergo an additional 2 years of training in a behavioral neurology fellowship. These physicians are experts in the field of dementia, specifically Alzheimer's, and treat complicated patients whose symptoms can sometimes extend beyond the scope of a general neurologist. Throughout the disease and diagnostic process, other medical specialties are called upon for their expertise. Radiologists, for example, play a significant role in imaging and the interpreting of scans. Additionally, if surgical intervention is deemed necessary or a patient has a concurrent brain bleed or tumor, neurological surgeons may sometimes play a role in the patient's treatment. Through the difficult journey of Alzheimer's, patients may find themselves interacting with multiple physicians with different fields of expertise in order to obtain a diagnosis and receive treatment.

As a first line of diagnosis, blood tests that specifically measure vitamin B12 levels, thyroid function, liver enzymes, and syphilis (a sexually transmitted disease that can lead to dementia) are performed. A derangement from normal of any of the tested values can be responsible for dementia and the cognitive findings. More recently, vitamin D deficiency has been shown to be related to dementia, but this relationship has not been fully elucidated and is not the standard of care at this time.

The next step in eliminating other potential causes of Alzheimer's disease is radiographic imaging of the brain. Physician's usually order non-contrast CT or MRI depending on their clinical suspicions. CT is better at determining any bleeds in the brain and MRI is better at viewing specific structures within the brain. Both imaging modalities highlight important features of the brain's anatomy and can be used to discover cerebral atrophy, one of the hallmarks of Alzheimer's disease. In cerebral atrophy, the brain becomes smaller and shrinks as a result of the disease process. Imaging studies show increased space between the brain and the skull, and larger ventricles. Despite this common finding, many other disease processes cause atrophy, and so this is non-diagnostic for Alzheimer's. Other imaging techniques that are still being debated include MRI of the hippocampus. Because the hippocampus plays an important role in memory, imaging it and determining its volume shows a sensitivity and specificity of 77% and 80% for Alzheimer's, respectively.[9] Sensitivity refers to the ability of the test to detect a disease when it is present, and specificity refers to the ability of the test to be "specific" to only that disease for which it is supposed to test and nothing else. Therefore, hippocampal imaging can detect Alzheimer's disease in 77% of patients that actually have Alzheimer's disease, but only 80% of patients with a positive test actually have Alzheimer's disease.

Other imaging modalities have also been used, such as single-photon emission computed tomography (SPECT) and positron emission tomography (PET). SPECT is useful in determining the blood flow to and oxygen in crucial parts of the brain in which disruption can cause dementia.[10] Nevertheless, these modalities are not commonly used in the normal work-up of Alzheimer's disease and are reserved for specific cases.

Lumbar punctures have also been shown to have limited utility in the diagnosis of Alzheimer's. A lumbar puncture (LP) consists of obtaining a sample of cerebrospinal fluid (CSF) from the patient. If the patient has too much CSF, as in hydrocephalus, the opening pressures (the pressure seen once the needle punctures the dura and is in the CSF space) will be high. Additionally, if infection is present, there will be makers of infection in the fluid (such as in dementia caused by syphilis). Today, experts argue about the use of lumbar punctures in patients with Alzheimer's disease. It has been shown that Alzheimer's patients have high levels of tau and phosphorylated tau, with correspondingly low amyloid levels. Although this has been proven as an approach to detecting Alzheimer's disease, doctors have no applicable therapy for reducing these proteins, and therefore this test does not change the management of the patient. For this reason, lumbar punctures are only deemed useful in a research setting rather than clinically.

Lastly, the genotyping of patients has become a test that can be used in patients with Alzheimer's disease. Genotyping is essentially a test that sequences the DNA of a patient and looks for specific genes that are responsible for coding specific proteins. One of these genes is called apolipoprotein E (*APOE*). *APOE*, specifically the *APOE-e4* variant of the gene, has been associated with an increased risk of developing amyloid deposits in the brain, which is one of the mechanisms of Alzheimer's disease. In this context, patients with the *APOE-e4* gene have an increased risk of developing Alzheimer's. Historically, genotyping has played no role in the clinical diagnosis of Alzheimer's and has been avoided in order to reduce unnecessary anxiety to patients who are deemed to be at increased risk for Alzheimer's, since no disease-altering treatments can be offered to patients.

Pathological findings

Plaques

Under a microscope, pathologists can clearly distinguish the differences between a normal brain and a brain that is afflicted with Alzheimer's disease. The hallmark pathological features of Alzheimer's disease include plaques, which are found outside the cells, and tangles, which are present within the cells. These abnormal proteins lead to an inflammatory response within the brain, just as a splinter or any foreign object would cause swelling and redness in the body. The inflammatory response contributes to the destructive tendencies of Alzheimer's disease, leading to a toxic environment within the brain and deteriorating the natural protective properties that the brain uses to protect itself

Differential Diagnosis for Dementia[11,12]

Disorder	Percentage of Dementia Cases	Key Symptoms	Pathological Findings	Method of Diagnosis
Alzheimer's disease	50–70%	Slow decrease in: — Memory — Normal function	β-amyloid plaques Tau tangles	Clinical diagnosis Neuropsychological evaluation Neurological examination (usually normal) Brain imaging (magnetic resonance imaging [MRI], positron emission tomography [PET]) Biomarkers (in the near future)
Vascular dementia	20%	"Post-stroke dementia" Symptoms depend on stroke location	Vascular damage Plaques Tangles	Brain Imaging (MRI, computed tomography)
Dementia with Lewy bodies (DLB)	10–25%	Fluctuation of: — Cognitive symptoms — Alertness — Visual hallucinations — Movement problems	Lewy bodies (composed of α-synuclein)	Brain imaging - (PET)~(MRI) Neuropsychological evaluation Neurological examination
Mixed dementia	10%	Combination of: — Alzheimer's — Other pathologies	Vascular damage Plaques Tangles	Brain imaging - (PET)~(MRI) Neuropsychological evaluation Neurological examination
Parkinson's disease (PD) dementia	2% of people >65 years of age	Problems with: — Movement (tremors, shakiness, stiffness, etc.)	Lewy bodies Loss of dopamine-producing neurons	Brain imaging (PET) Neurological examination
Frontotemporal dementia (FTD) or Pick's disease	Rare	Changes in: — Behavior/personality — Writing — Understanding	Tau TDP43 (a specific protein)	Brain imaging - (PET)~(MRI) Neuropsychological evaluation Neurological examination

Disease	Frequency	Symptoms	Brain findings	Diagnosis
Creutzfeldt–Jakob disease	Rare (1 in 1 million people)	Rapid decline in: — Thinking — Reasoning	Sponge-like lesions in the brain	Brain imaging (MRI), Lumbar puncture, Electroencephalogram (EEG)
Other mimickers of dementia				
Mild cognitive impairment (MCI)	MCI is not dementia (can progress to dementia)	Normal cognition, Mild memory deficits	Sometimes seen: — β-amyloid plaques — Tau tangles	Clinical diagnosis, Neuropsychological evaluation, Neurological examination
Depression	Very common (seen in 12.7% of Alzheimer's patients)[13]	Symptoms mimic Alzheimer's disease, Low energy, Apathetic	None	Psychiatric evaluation (Geriatric Depression Scale used for screening)
Normal pressure hydrocephalus	Very common	Difficulty with: — Walking — Thinking — Bladder control	Enlarged ventricles	Brain imaging - (PET)~(MRI), Neurological examination, Lumbar puncture
Huntington's disease	Genetic (50% chance of developing if familial)	Involuntary movements, Changes in: — Memory — Personality — Balance	Mutation causes degeneration of nerve cells	Genetic testing, Brain imaging - (PET)~(MRI), Neurological examination
Wernicke–Korsakoff syndrome	Uncommon, Increases risk of Alzheimer's	Confusion, Confabulation, Unsteadiness	Vitamin B1 deficiency	Laboratory tests (blood test)
Vitamin B12 deficiency	Very common	Balance problems, Weakness, Numbness	Vitamin B12 deficiency	Laboratory tests (blood test)
Infection (encephalitis, meningitis)	Common	Lethargy, Cognitive deterioration	White blood cells seen in cerebrospinal fluid	Lumbar puncture

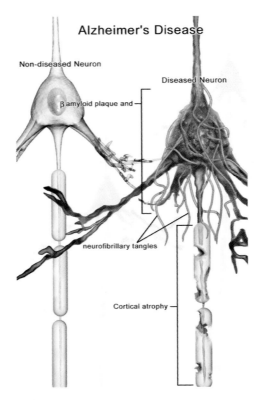

Fig. 5.2.   The hallmark plaques and tangles found in Alzheimer's disease. (Figure credit: Ref. 14.)

from damage. However, the presence of these proteins in the brain usually indicates the later stages of a disease process that has been present for some time.

The senile plaques found in the brains of Alzheimer's disease patients are composed of small protein subunits known as β-amyloid. The β-amyloid fragments are actually created by the enzymatic processing of a larger protein known as amyloid precursor protein, or APP for short. APP is normally found in the membranes of neurons and has normal regulatory functions in the cell. When it is cleaved by two separate enzymes known as β- and γ-secretase, the resulting β-amyloid fragments accumulate and form plaques. These plaques are extremely disruptive

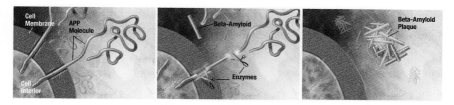

Fig. 5.3. Enzymes (β- and γ-secretase) cleave the amyloid precursor protein (APP) into small protein fragments. These fragments can include the β-amyloid fragment, which can self-link to form oligomers (many fragments linked together) and eventually fibrils (many oligomers linked together) that result in plaques. (Figure credit: Ref. 15.)

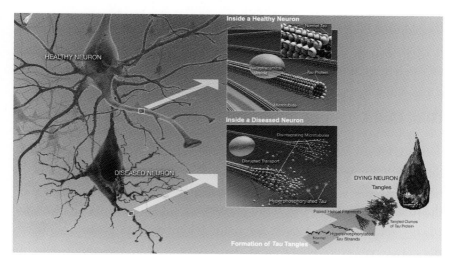

Fig. 5.4. Depiction of tau tangle formation. (Figure credit: Ref. 16.)

to normal cellular processes and communication and contribute to the death of neurons in Alzheimer's disease.

Tangles

In addition to the plaques, neurofibrillary tangles are a prominent pathological feature of Alzheimer's disease. The tangles are aggregates of a protein known as tau. This tau protein becomes "hyperphosphorylated," meaning that too many phosphate molecules are added to the protein.

When tau is hyperphosphorylated, it forms an insoluble twisted fiber within the neuron. This tangle disrupts normal nutrient transport and cellular functioning, leading to cell death.

Cerebral Amyloid Angiopathy

In addition to the plaques and tangles that are characteristic of Alzheimer's disease, other changes also occur. These include something known as cerebral amyloid angiopathy, which is a blood vessel abnormality in which amyloid deposits accrue in the walls of the blood vessels within the central nervous system. Cerebral amyloid angiopathy can actually increase the risk of bleeding within the brain, and also increases the risk of developing dementia when present in isolation.[17]

Glial Cell Changes

The brains of individuals with Alzheimer's disease exhibit a prolific glial cell response. The glial cells in the brain are important mediators of inflammation.[18] The activation of a specific group of glial cells that destroy other cells in the brain (cytotoxic; *cyto* means "cell" and *toxic* means "harmful") has even been linked to neurodegenerative disorders. Two particular glial cells that are important in Alzheimer's disease pathology are astrocytes and microglial cells. These cells are commonly found near the β-amyloid plaques in the brain, and are activated by or react to the plaques.[19]

Astrocytes play an important role in the brain because they are actually involved in the accumulation of β-amyloid and, specifically, β-amyloid 42 (Aβ42), which is the protein that is specific to Alzheimer's disease. When astrocytes are "overburdened" with too much Aβ42, they can burst open and dispel their contents into the surrounding cells, which can contribute to the formation of β-amyloid plaques.

The microglia, on the other hand, are more involved in the inflammatory response in the brain. Microglial cells are actually derived from a specific type of white blood cell known as a macrophage, which is an important immune cell in the body. When plaques are present in the brain, the microglia migrate to the location of the microscopic plaques, leading to morphological changes in the plaques. This change is very important because it transforms the soluble β-amyloid fragments into insoluble plaques. Therefore, the blockade of Aβ42 accumulation within neurons and astrocytes, as well as the inhibition of microglia, may be potential therapeutic targets.[20]

Neuronal and Synaptic Loss

The previously discussed pathological changes that are present in Alzheimer's disease are known as "positive changes," since they are additional features that are not seen in normal brain tissue. In addition to these positive changes, there are some negative changes that are associated with Alzheimer's disease. As can be inferred from the term, negative changes refer to things that are not present in Alzheimer's disease brains when compared to normal brains. The major "negative" pathological changes seen in Alzheimer's disease are the loss of neurons and the loss of synaptic connections.

The loss of neurons is due to the widespread apoptosis (pre-programmed cell death) throughout the brain due to the destructive and damaging properties of the plaques, tangles, glial cell response, and amyloid deposition within the brain. The apoptosis, as mentioned previously, leads to a macroscopic change known as atrophy, or overall shrinkage of the brain tissue. In addition to neuronal apoptosis, there is an accompanying loss of synaptic connections in the brain. Interestingly, studies performed at autopsy in patients of different ages have shown that the build-up of amyloid plaques in the brain actually precedes the onset of cognitive deterioration in patients with Alzheimer's disease. This is in contrast to the presence of neurofibrillary tangles, as well as neuronal and synaptic loss, which are actually directly correlated and "parallel" the cognitive deterioration seen in Alzheimer's disease.

The findings of these autopsy studies have been confirmed with modern imaging techniques such as PET scans that can monitor amyloid deposits in live humans.[21]

Now that we have discussed the microscopic pathological changes that occur in Alzheimer's disease, let us explore the macroscopic changes that are visible to the naked eye.

Macroscopic Changes

If one were to observe the brain of an Alzheimer's patient, it would be fairly different from a normal brain in many respects. First, the overall damage caused by Alzheimer's disease kills many cells within the brain — this eventually leads to the brain shrinking in size, or atrophy. This atrophy can sometimes lead to an increase in the size of the ventricles within the brain. As we discussed in the first chapter of this book, the ventricles are basically reservoirs of a watery substance known as CSF. If the ventricles increase in size due to global brain atrophy, the amount of CSF that needs to be produced increases. Unfortunately, as individuals age, CSF production decreases, and this decrease in CSF production is exacerbated by Alzheimer's disease.[22] The decreased production of CSF leads to a decrease in the filtration of the toxic proteins and molecules that accumulate in the brain.[23,24] Furthermore, the decreased production of CSF is complemented by decreased reabsorption of CSF. This leads to a reduction in the overall turnover of CSF in the brain, and can cause ventricular enlargement. Unfortunately, the decrease in CSF turnover also increases the toxic amyloid proteins in the brain and may contribute to the formation of neuronal plaques.

In addition to the decrease in the overall size of the brain, the grooves that are normally found on the brain surface (they serve to increase the overall surface area) increase in size. Interestingly, in Alzheimer's disease, there is a disproportionate loss of brain tissue on the sides of the brain, specifically referred to as the temporal regions of brain. In particular, the area of the Sylvian fissure (see Fig. 5.5), also known as the

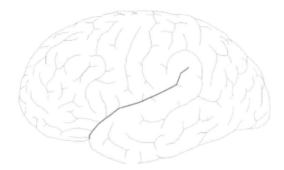

Fig. 5.5.   The Sylvian fissure (also known as the lateral sulcus) is highlighted in red. This region of the brain is disproportionately atrophied in Alzheimer's disease. (Figure credit: Ref. 25.)

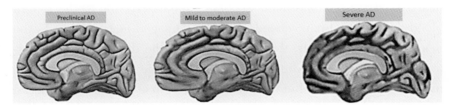

Fig. 5.6.   As Alzheimer's disease progresses from the region of the hippocampus (which is located deep within the temporal lobes of the brain), the atrophy (cell death) becomes more pronounced and affects the entire brain. (Modified from Ref. 26.)

lateral sulcus, exhibits significant neuronal loss and atrophy. This leads to the characteristic gross (macroscopic) shrunken appearance of an Alzheimer's brain.

Cause of Death

Interestingly, the cause of death from Alzheimer's disease is not actually directly due to the disease process itself. Normally, the cause of death is due to a complication that arises due to the disease process. In two-thirds of Alzheimer's patients, the cause of death is pneumonia; however, other causes, such as respiratory depression or sepsis (infection), may also contribute. The pneumonia is usually due to the suppression of the cough reflex by the disease. The cough reflex is particularly important in preventing aspiration pneumonia, which is pneumonia that is caused by a foreign substance or fluid being inhaled into the lungs. Individuals with Alzheimer's disease are cognitively impaired to the point that the cough reflex does not properly function. Additionally, problems with swallowing and chewing due to the disease can eventually lead to food and fluid being aspirated into the lungs, causing pneumonia.

Natural History

The term "natural history" refers to the course of a disease process when left untreated. For example, if an individual were to have a massive heart attack, they would likely become unconscious due to the lack of blood flow to the brain secondary to the damaged heart tissue. As the heart damage manifests, that individual may die due to a lack of systemic blood flow, or perfusion. This would be the natural history of an untreated heart attack, but if we modify the course of a disease process, as in the case of providing cardiopulmonary resuscitation, emergency cardiac bypass surgery, or administering medications that improve the cardiovascular system, the individual may eventually survive the heart attack. Alzheimer's disease is one of the few diseases in which the natural history of the disease process is relatively unchanged and, at best, mildly attenuated by modern treatments.

The natural course of a patient suffering from Alzheimer's disease progresses from mild cognitive changes initially, through a series of steps that eventually leads to a near-vegetative state and death. Alzheimer's disease can generally be broken up into an early, middle, and late stage (see Table 5.3).

In the early stages, the hallmark features are cognitive changes, including memory loss, personality changes, agitation, and a myriad of other behavioral alterations. As the disease progresses into the middle stages, the cognitive changes worsen and begin to significantly impact the patient's normal everyday activities, or activities of daily

Table 5.3. Symptoms of Alzheimer's Disease by Stage[27]

Early stage	Middle stage	Late stage
• Word-finding difficulties • Difficulty remembering names of new people • Difficulty with social and work tasks • Forgetting recently read material • Misplacing valuable objects • Difficulty planning or organizing	• Forgetting important events or personal memories • Moodiness or social withdrawal • Inability to recall address or telephone numbers • Confusion with dates and location • Difficulty selecting proper clothing • Bladder and bowel incontinence • Sleep pattern changes • Risk of wandering or being lost • Personality or behavioral changes (suspicion, impulsiveness, delusions, and repetitive behaviors)	• Need full-time assistance required for activities of daily living • No awareness of recent and past experiences or surroundings • Deterioration of physical capabilities, including walking, sitting, and eventually swallowing • Communication problems • Vulnerability to pneumonia and infection

living (ADL). This results in significant stress to both the patient and his or her caregivers. The amount of time and effort that is required in order to care for the patient's everyday needs is tremendous, and families often face extremely difficult social and financial hardships as they struggle to find the time and energy to care for their loved ones. For example, many caregivers must take significant time away from their careers in order to focus on caring for their family member with Alzheimer's disease. This can lead to significant financial strains on caregivers and families.

The unrelenting progression of the disease eventually leads to the late stages of Alzheimer's disease. This stage is signified by a nearly complete loss of the patient's ability to care for themselves; from eating and swallowing to using the restroom and dressing themselves, patients in the late stages of Alzheimer's disease are tremendously impaired, and it is during this time that the patient and their family face some of the most difficult hardships. All cognitive abilities, including speech, are permanently destroyed. The personality and behaviors that once defined the individual are no longer present, and in their place, a vegetative body remains.

The pathology and progression of Alzheimer's disease is unrelenting and horrendous. In classical Alzheimer's disease, fewer than 3% of individuals survive 14 years after they are initially diagnosed. The amount of time that individuals survive after diagnosis is dependent on a variety of factors. Confounding factors, such as developing a urinary tract infection, pneumonia, or other medical conditions, can accelerate cognitive decline and more profoundly affect Alzheimer's patients than normal healthy patients. This is due to a decrease in resilience in the brains and overall physiological functioning of patients with Alzheimer's disease. The difficulties in treating the disease have made it extremely interesting and compelling to study, yet mysterious and tortuous in terms of discovering what is truly going on within the brains of Alzheimer's patients and how we can fix them.

References

1. http://www.alz.org/facts/overview.asp

2. http://www.alz.org/boomers/

3. https://upload.wikimedia.org/wikipedia/commons/a/a5/Alzheimer%27s_disease_brain_comparison.jpg

4. http://www.webmd.com/alzheimers/news/20040405/alzheimers-disease-predicting-survival

5. Teng E, Ringman JM, Ross LK, *et al.* (2008) Diagnosing depression in Alzheimer disease with the National Institute of Mental Health provisional criteria. *Am J Geriatr Psychiatry* **16**(6): 469–477.

6. Vann Jones SA, O'Brien JT. (2014) The prevalence and incidence of dementia with Lewy bodies: A systematic review of population and clinical studies. *Psychol Med* **44**(4): 673–683.

7. Geser F, Wenning GK, Poewe W, McKeith I. (2005) How to diagnose dementia with Lewy bodies: State of the art. *Movement Disord* **20**(Suppl. 12): S11–S20.

8. Osimani A, Berger A, Friedman J, *et al.* (2005) Neuropsychology of vitamin B12 deficiency in elderly dementia patients and control subjects. *J Geriatr Psychiatry Neurol* **18**(1): 33–38.

9. Jack CR Jr, Petersen RC, Xu YC, *et al.* (1997) Medial temporal atrophy on MRI in normal aging and very mild Alzheimer's disease. *Neurology* **49**(3): 786–794.

10. DeKosky ST, Shih WJ, Schmitt FA, *et al.* (1990) Assessing utility of single photon emission computed tomography (SPECT) scan in Alzheimer disease: Correlation with cognitive severity. *Alzheimer Dis Assoc Disord* **4**(1): 14–23.

11. http://www.alz.org/dementia/types-of-dementia.asp

12. http://www.alz.org/professionals_and_researchers_13507.asp

13. Chi S, Wang C, Jiang T, *et al.* (2015) The prevalence of depression in Alzheimer's disease: A systematic review and meta-analysis. *Curr Alzheimer Res* **12**(2): 189–198.

14. https://commons.wikimedia.org/wiki/File:Blausen_0017_Alzheimers Disease.png

15. https://commons.wikimedia.org/wiki/File:Alzheimers_disease-Beta-amyloid_plaque_formation.PNG

16. https://commons.wikimedia.org/wiki/File:Tau_tangle_formation.jpg

17. https://www.nlm.nih.gov/medlineplus/ency/article/000719.htm

18. Von Bernhardi R. (2007) Glial cell dysregulation: a new perspective on Alzheimer disease. *Neurotox Res* **12**(4): 215–232.

19. Meda L, Baron P, Scarlato G. (2001) Glial activation in Alzheimer's disease: The role of Aβ and its associated proteins. *Neurobiol Aging* **22**(6): 885–893.

20. Nagele RG, Wegiel J, Venkataraman V, *et al.* (2004) Contribution of glial cells to the development of amyloid plaques in Alzheimer's disease. *Neurobiol Aging* **25**(5): 663–674.

21. http://perspectivesinmedicine.cshlp.org/content/1/1/a006189.full

22. Chen CPC, Chen RL, Preston JE. (2010) The influence of cerebrospinal fluid turnover on age-related changes in cerebrospinal fluid protein concentrations. *Neurosci Lett* **476**(3): 138–141.

23. Garton MJ, Keir G, Lakshmi MV, Thompson EJ. (1991) Age-related changes in cerebrospinal fluid protein concentrations. *J Neurol Sci* **104**(1): 74–80.

24. Kawarabayashi T, Younkin LH, Saido TC, *et al.* (2001) Age-dependent changes in brain, CSF, and plasma amyloid β protein in the Tg2576 transgenic mouse model of Alzheimer's disease. *J Neurosci* **21**(2): 372–381.

25. https://commons.wikimedia.org/wiki/Category:Lateral_sulcus#/media/File:Lateral_sulcus.png

26. https://commons.wikimedia.org/wiki/File:Alzheimers_disease_progression-brain_degeneration.PNG

27. http://www.alz.org/alzheimers_disease_stages_of_alzheimers.asp

Chapter 6

Epidemiology of Alzheimer's Disease

"As our world continues to generate unimaginable amounts of data, more data lead to more correlations, and more correlations can lead to more discoveries."

— Hans Rosling, Professor of International Health, Karolinska Institute

Alzheimer's disease is extremely prevalent and pervasive within our society. It truly is a disease that almost every individual in the country is aware of, and one that has personally affected millions of Americans. However, in order to ensure that all readers are up-to-date on the epidemiology of Alzheimer's disease, let us walk through some important points related to Alzheimer's disease.

Alzheimer's disease is the most common form of dementia, has no cure and no effective treatment, and always leads to death. Alzheimer's disease is commonly diagnosed in individuals over 65 years of age, and the prevalence of the disease increases as individuals get older. Although Alzheimer's disease is classically considered to be a disease of elderly individuals, this is not always the case. There is a rare form of Alzheimer's disease, known as early-onset Alzheimer's disease, which affects certain individuals in as early as their third and fourth decades of life.[1] Early-onset Alzheimer's disease makes up approximately 5% of all Alzheimer's patients. This is a devastating age to be diagnosed with a disease that tears apart the mind at such a productive age. Although some individuals diagnosed in their 30s and 40s are able to live fruitful lives for several years after diagnosis, relatively few survive into their 50s and 60s. As previously mentioned, less than 3% of patients with Alzheimer's disease survive 14 years after they are initially diagnosed. In addition to this meager life expectancy, the corresponding deterioration in the patient's quality of life is stark. The disease process is unrelenting and unbiased in whom it targets. Alzheimer's disease affects individuals from all socioeconomic backgrounds, from grandparents or football players, to presidents (Ronald Reagan) and Nobel Laureates (Charles Kao).

However, new evidence is suggesting that some individuals are at an increased risk compared with others. It has recently been demonstrated that football players who have experienced repeated blows to the head have a higher prevalence of Alzheimer's disease in addition to other neurodegenerative disorders, such as amyotrophic lateral sclerosis (ALS).[2] With repeated blows to the head, the body responds by creating inflammation, more specifically called neuroinflammation. This neuroinflammation activates various repair cells, such as microglial and astroglial cells (see Chapter 5). Although these cells attempt to fix the injury, they unfortunately are the cause of the post-traumatic neurodegeneration that ensues. This can subsequently contribute to the development of Alzheimer's disease.

Gender and Ethnicity

Interestingly, gender may also play a role in Alzheimer's disease. Although not fully accepted by experts, one study found that women have a twofold increase in Alzheimer's disease risk compared with men.[3] This is interesting because men have actually been shown to have a higher risk of developing mild cognitive impairment (MCI), which is a middle ground between normal brain function and dementia.[4] The reason for this is unclear; however, differences in brain size, brain function, genetics, hormones, and social differences between the genders have been postulated to play a role.

Brain Size and Function

Men classically have larger brain volumes, while women have increased synaptic density.[5] Women also have a larger amount of grey matter in their brains (which is composed of neuronal cell bodies) and men have a larger percentage of white matter (composed of myelinated axons).[6,7] Furthermore, differences in blood flow to the brain, synaptic connectivity, and metabolic deficits may play a role in why women are more likely to develop Alzheimer's disease.[8] One theory even postulates that regions of the brain with higher synaptic connections may be more prone to developing plaques, thus making women more susceptible to these plaques.[9]

Genetics

Genetically, the *APOE-e4* allele has even been shown to have more pronounced effects in women than in men, and some studies have suggested that the presence of the allele in women results in a fourfold increased risk of Alzheimer's disease, while men with the allele only had mildly increased risk.[10,11] Another gene, known as the brain-derived neurotrophic factor (*BDNF*) gene, was found to be associated with an increased risk of developing Alzheimer's disease only in women, but not in men.[12] Another genetic factor that may play a role is known as single-nucleotide polymorphisms (SNPs). SNPs are isolated changes in a single part of the genome, and can sometimes be associated with certain disease states. However, certain SNPs have been found to increase the risk of Alzheimer's disease in men instead of women, while others were found to have exactly the opposite effect.[13,14]

Hormones

In addition to genetic factors, hormonal factors may play a role in the gender discrepancies in Alzheimer's disease. After menopause, women have a decrease in certain sex hormones, such as progesterone and estradiol.[15] Men also have a 2–3% decrease in testosterone levels annually after 30 years of age, but this decline is more gradual.[16] Furthermore, testosterone can be metabolized into estrogen, and therefore men have lower levels of estrogen loss in later life. Estrogen has been shown to be neuroprotective and can improve synaptic formation, hippocampal function, blood flow, and glucose metabolism in the brain, improved synthesis of acetylcholine (an important neurotransmitter in Alzheimer's disease and normal memory), and can prevent mitochondrial damage.[17-23] Despite these findings, the roles of estrogen, and even hormone-replacement therapy (HRT) for restoring low levels of estrogen in women, have been unclear.[24-28]

One study conducted at the Mayo Clinic investigated women who had their ovaries removed prior to menopause. They found that these women had a nearly twofold increase in the risk of dementia.[29] Interestingly, the study found that in women who were started on HRT following surgery to remove their ovaries, there was no increased risk of Alzheimer's disease. However, a large study known as the Women's Health Initiative Memory Study (WHIMS) found that women who were started on HRT after the age of 65 had a twofold increased risk of developing dementia.[30] The reason for these disparate results is unclear; however, it may relate to the timing of the delivery of the HRT.[31] It has been proposed that when HRT is initiated within 5 years of women developing menopause rather than many years later, the risk of developing Alzheimer's disease is decreased by up to 30%. But when HRT is initiated 5 years after the development of menopause or after the age of 65, there was actually a twofold increase in the risk of developing Alzheimer's disease.

The biological explanation for why estrogen can have an effect on the development of Alzheimer's disease is unclear. However, one hypothesis states that long-term estrogen depletion (LTED) can lead to decreased levels of a particular estrogen receptor (estrogen receptor-α) in the hippocampus. If estrogen depletion leads to less estrogen receptors over time, the addition of estrogen via HRT may not have a beneficial effect.[32] Another hypothesis states that estrogen can only be neuroprotective when the neurons are healthy.[33] When neurons are damaged, as in the case of Alzheimer's disease and with aging, the beneficial effects of estrogen can actually become harmful.

Social and Behavioral Effects

In addition to the biological differences between men and women that may underlie the differences in their risk of developing Alzheimer's disease, social factors such as education, occupation, exercise, diet, smoking, alcohol consumption, and cognitive activity may also be contributory. In fact, these factors can contribute up to 10% of the divergence in cognitive performance in individuals.[34] Education and occupational history have been linked to Alzheimer's disease, with cognitive stimulation protecting against dementia.[35-45] Interestingly, decreased cognitive performance and IQ in the early years of life are associated with decreased cognitive function in later years, as well as increased dementia and mortality risk.[46-48] Brain imaging has even shown that individuals who have more educational or work experience have the same cognitive performance on tasks as individuals with fewer abnormalities in their brains.[49-52] The reason for this may be explained by the finding that individuals with more education have higher initial cognitive functioning in comparison with individuals with less education, and can therefore appear normal for a longer time prior to being diagnosed with dementia.[53] Furthermore, societal influences have traditionally provided men with more higher-educational opportunities in the 20th century, and could lead to higher cognitive reserve in males, which could impact the gender difference in Alzheimer's disease prevalence. Women have also been shown to be more cognitively engaged in daily activities such as reading, hobbies, and social activities, which could improve their cognitive reserve, but not to the same degree as educational and occupational history.

In addition to education, exercise is another behavioral factor that can affect dementia risk. It is well established that cardiovascular health, which is highly predicated upon a proper exercise and diet regimen, is highly correlated with MCI and Alzheimer's disease.[54–58] Interestingly, marital status and being a parent can negatively impact the amount of exercise that women get, and women on average participate in less exercise than men throughout their lives.[59,60] However, studies have produced conflicting data regarding whether or not there are differences in the effects of exercise on Alzheimer's risk in women compared to men. It seems that exercise is helpful regardless of gender, with no confirmed additional positive or negative impact of exercise on women compared to men.[61–63] One thing that has become clear, however, is that exercise in the teenage years is associated with the greatest reduction in dementia risk. The importance of exercise cannot be understated. Regardless of age, exercise is beneficial and protective against a host of medical disorders, but in addition to a healthy exercise regimen, other behavioral factors such as diet, smoking, alcohol consumption, and more can influence the development of Alzheimer's disease.

Smoking

A report by the Centers for Disease Control and Prevention (CDC) showed that in 2013, 15.3% of women and 20.5% of men smoked in the USA.[64] In 1965, this number was 33.9% in women and 51.9% in men. Studies have shown that male smokers have an increased risk of developing Alzheimer's disease compared with female smokers.[65] Smoking is an important risk factor for the development of cardiovascular disease, cancer, dementia, and many other medical diseases. However, smoking has very interesting effects that are particularly relevant in Alzheimer's disease. Cigarette smoke contains high levels of nicotine, which can activate a specific class of receptors that are decreased in Alzheimer's disease (specifically known as nicotinic acetylcholine receptors). At first, scientists thought that since the nicotine in cigarettes could activate these downregulated receptors in Alzheimer's disease, then perhaps smoking could decrease the risk of Alzheimer's. Furthermore, studies have shown that nicotine has positive cognitive effects in humans.[66] This actually led to the development of a clinical trial in which nicotine patches were tested in Alzheimer's disease patients. However, these trials have produced mixed results, with some indicating cognitive protection and others showing no effect.[67,68] Despite these findings, cigarette smoke contains hundreds of harmful chemicals that can increase the risk of developing Alzheimer's disease, cancer, heart disease, and lung disease. Smoking can be even more damaging when combined with heavy alcohol use, and studies have shown that heavy drinkers who also smoked had a quicker decline in cognitive function than those who abstained.[69]

In animals, cigarette smoke has been shown to be very damaging to neurons and the brain. Cigarette smoke has been shown to result in amyloid deposition in the brain, phosphorylation of the tau protein (the important protein that is involved in Alzheimer's disease), inflammation and decreased oxygen levels within the brain, and neurodegeneration.[70,71] In humans, smoking has been shown to increase brain atrophy and increase the risk of developing Alzheimer's disease.[72–75]

Ethnicity

In addition to gender, Alzheimer's disease has also been seen to have different prevalence rates between ethnicities. Studies have found that African–Americans exhibit higher instances of dementias in general — they are twice as likely to have Alzheimer's disease. Additionally, Hispanics are 1.5-times more likely to develop Alzheimer's disease compared to Caucasians. Other racial groups have not been studied in sufficiently large groups to draw statistically significant conclusions.

The reason for the differences in the prevalence rates of Alzheimer's disease between individuals of various ethnic groups is multifactorial. One link that has been studied is genetic. In a genome-wide association study (GWAS) — a study type that examines the entire genetic code in all participants for possible genetic similarities that could explain a disease process — the *APOE-e4* allele and the *ABCA7* gene were found to be related to an increased risk of Alzheimer's disease in African–Americans.[76] In addition to genetic factors, medical conditions such as diabetes and high blood pressure are more common in African–Americans and Hispanics than in Caucasians. These medical conditions may increase the likelihood of developing Alzheimer's disease and dementia. Studies investigating the link between socioeconomic factors and Alzheimer's disease found that when all factors (such as education and income) were equal, there was no dramatic increase in Alzheimer's risk.

Global Effects

There are over 30 million people suffering from Alzheimer's disease in the world, and it has been projected that 1 in 85 individuals will be diagnosed with Alzheimer's disease by 2050. As of 2014, there have been over 1,500 clinical trials that have been conducted or are being conducted on Alzheimer's disease. Unfortunately, none of them has been able to cure the disease.

The Alzheimer's Association website writes in bold: "Invest in a world without Alzheimer's." What would this world look like? We would have the ability to treat the majority of the 46.8 million people currently living in the world with dementia as of 2015 — an estimated 22.9 million in Asia, 10.5 million in Europe, 9.4 million in the Americas, and 4.0 million in Africa. We would save 17.9 billion extra hours if we cured American citizens alone, hours that have been contributed by friends and family members of Alzheimer's patients in unpaid care. We would be a world that would be richer by $818 billion US dollars, which is the amount that dementia has cost us in 2015 alone.[77] From 2010 to 2015, annual costs per person for the treatment of Alzheimer's vary across the world, ranging from $872 (South Asia) to $56,218 (North America). There are steps being taken towards global action and unity by countries and regions around the world in order to understand, stop, and ultimately treat Alzheimer's disease. This makes sense — dementia is a global problem, so action should be taken in the same vein.

One research study conducted by Professor Martin Prince and his colleagues[78] found that, across the world, the age-standardized prevalence rate of dementia is 5–7%. They conducted a systematic review of all published literature around the world on the prevalence of dementia from between 1980 and 2009. They then conducted a meta-analysis (a large statistical analysis) in order to estimate the prevalence of individuals aged 60 or older with dementia. Interestingly, they found a higher prevalence of dementia in Latin America (8.5%) and a lower prevalence in sub-Saharan African regions (2–4%). They estimated that approximately 35.6 million people lived with dementia worldwide in 2010, and proposed that this number would be expected to double every 20 years. They found that 58% of individuals living with dementia were in countries with low or middle incomes, and they expected this proportion to rise to 71% by 2050. In the USA alone, an estimated 5.3 million individuals have Alzheimer's disease (in 2015), with 200,000 individuals with early- or younger-onset Alzheimer's (below the age of 65).[79]

As per the Alzheimer's World Report 2015, a decline in the age-specific incidence of dementia is possible, at least in high-income countries, fueled by awareness of the risk factors for dementia, such as lifestyle and cardiovascular changes. Thus, it appears that the future path of the Alzheimer's epidemic is likely to be influenced by efforts to improve public health such as preventing, detecting, and controlling obesity, hypertension, and diabetes in order to improve brain health.[80] Although high-income countries have been focusing their efforts on aging, dementia, and Alzheimer's, it is speculated that the global burden of the disease will shift inexorably to low- and middle-income countries in the next few decades, with 71% of those with dementia living in lower- and middle-income countries by 2050. To make matters worse, most leaders — of nations and public health organizations alike — have underestimated the global burden of Alzheimer's up until now. For example, a

2010 *Lancet* study reported that China had more people living with Alzheimer's disease than any other country in the world, and twice as many cases of Alzheimer's and other kinds of dementia as the World Health Organization (WHO) speculated.[81]

Professor Martin Prince from King's College London, author of *The Global Impact of Dementia 2013–2050*, says that dementia will impact "developing countries with limited resources and little time to develop comprehensive systems of social protection, health, and social care." A key note from the above Policy Brief, written in preparation for the 2013 G8 Dementia Summit, is to learn from the HIV epidemic regarding the importance of well-established care systems and access to diagnostic technologies and drug therapies in low- and middle-income countries. In an effort to enable international action for addressing dementia, health ministers who are part of the Alzheimer's Disease International (ADI) organization met in December 2013 for the G8 Dementia Summit in London. As of 2013, only 13 out of the 193 WHO countries have national dementia plans in place.[82] As per the Summit's declaration, there are plans for cross-country partnerships and efforts, focusing on: (1) social impact investment (UK led); (2) new care and prevention models (Japan led); and (3) academia–industry partnerships (Canada and France co-led). The G8 countries also emphasized the need for all countries — not just the ones participating — to contribute to these international plans.[83]

An important point that came out of the G8 Summit was encouraging open access to data and thus accelerating research and solutions for Alzheimer's disease. In early fall of 2015, a platform for open access was becoming a reality with the launching of the Global Alzheimer's Association Interactive Network (GAAIN), an open-access, big-data online platform for coordinating the global collaboration of Alzheimer's disease research. The GAAIN initiative is planned to be completed in 5 years. The first phase of its development involves designing a query infrastructure, integrating the data networks of GAAIN partners, and providing a user-friendly interface.

The International Alzheimer's Disease Research Portfolio (IADRP), developed by the National Institute on Aging (NIA), part of the National Institutes of Health (NIH), in collaboration with the Alzheimer's Association will enable public and private funders of Alzheimer's research to coordinate research planning, leverage resources, avoid duplication of funding efforts, and identify new opportunities in promising areas of growth.[84]

There is still a long way to go, but ideas for an effective, coordinated international response to Alzheimer's are in the pipeline. The next G8 Summit will be held in the USA in May 2016 to review progress. This is a very small piece of the global story of the fight against Alzheimer's, and volumes more could be written on the global response to Alzheimer's disease. However, let us focus on the USA's efforts to stop the progression of Alzheimer's as an example of a country's response to a debilitating illness.

National Effects

Alzheimer's disease is the sixth leading cause of death in the USA. Due to the impact it has on the patient and their family members, it creates a disproportionately large economic burden on the USA, costing over $226,000,000,000 ($226 billion) per year.[85] This is a sixth of the national defense budget and seven-times more than the entire NIH budget for medical research annually ($30.1 billion).[86]

The war against Alzheimer's disease has just begun, and we are beginning to develop the appropriate tools and acquire the necessary understanding of both normal and abnormal brain functioning in order to adequately address the elimination of Alzheimer's disease. Although the most dramatic effects of Alzheimer's disease are seen when considering the afflicted individual and their friends and family, the damaging effects of the disease extend far beyond the family. Alzheimer's disease affects all aspects of society. From politics to economics, it takes a substantive toll. One of the more influential political figures in recent history was Ronald Reagan, who famously was diagnosed and eventually died while having Alzheimer's disease. The deterioration of a once-powerful world figure into complete cognitive vegetation highlighted the devastation that Alzheimer's causes, and brought this disease into the national spotlight.

Despite a major political figure falling victim to Alzheimer's disease, one of the major shortfalls when it comes to Alzheimer's research is a lack of federal funding. The US government spends $562 million on Alzheimer's disease annually, despite the fact that the disease costs the USA $226 billion a year.[87] In fact, every dollar spent on Alzheimer's research could be considered an investment in the future thanks to the economic costs saved when patients and their families are able to contribute to society in a meaningful way, rather than being sequestered in their homes.[88] For comparison, a 2011 report by Battelle showed that "the NIH-led Human Genome Project generated a staggering return on investment of $141 for every dollar spent on the project."[89] According to a testimony by Harry Johns, President and CEO of the Alzheimer's Association, presented to the US House of Representatives in 2014, "For every $31,000 Medicare and Medicaid spends caring for individuals with Alzheimer's, the NIH spends only $100 on Alzheimer's research."[90] Furthermore, a publication titled *Changing the Trajectory of Alzheimer's Disease: How a Treatment by 2025 Saves Lives and Dollars* by the Alzheimer's Association states:

> "...a treatment introduced in 2025 that delays the onset of Alzheimer's by five years would reduce the number of individuals affected by the disease immediately. In 2030, the total number of Americans age 65 and older living with Alzheimer's would decrease from 8.2 million to 5.8 million ... In 2035, 4 million Americans — approximately 40 percent of the 9.9 million Americans who would be expected to have Alzheimer's — would be living without it. In 2050, total prevalence would be 7.8 million, meaning 5.7 million Americans — or 42 percent of the 13.5 million who would be

expected to have Alzheimer's barring a treatment breakthrough — would not have Alzheimer's disease." These statistics are extremely motivating as a breakthrough in the treatment of Alzheimer's that would simply delay its onset would be hugely beneficial for patients, caregivers, and the nation as a whole."

The fact that Alzheimer's disease not only affects the livelihood and productivity of the individual who is afflicted with the disease, but also an entire network of family and friends surrounding that patient, highlights the significant economic impact that the disease has. In order to tackle a problem of such magnitude, governmental involvement in the form of grants and funding for various educational and caregiver assistance programs is necessary.

The national government, specifically the NIA — a branch of the NIH — recognizes the public health impact of Alzheimer's disease. The NIA was created by Congress in 1974 in order to facilitate research, training, and educational programs pertaining to aging and seniors. Future amendments eventually designated the NIA as the primary federal agency of Alzheimer's disease research.[91] With this came many advancements towards understanding and caring for patients with Alzheimer's. In 1984, the first Alzheimer's disease centers are established. In 2003, the NIA in collaboration with the Alzheimer's Association developed the Alzheimer's Disease Genetics Initiative in order to create a large bank of genetic materials, cell lines, and data from families so as to accelerate the discovery of the genes involved in late-onset Alzheimer's disease.[92] At its outset, Alzheimer's disease centers, NIA-supported researchers across the USA, and the Alzheimer's Association's network of local chapters recruited families with multiple members diagnosed with late-onset Alzheimer's disease in order to collect samples and supporting data from 1,000 families over a 3-year period. We can see the joint efforts of the national government and public organizations coming together in order to maximize the discovery and sharing of information. In fact, the National Alzheimer's Project Act (NAPA) was passed unanimously by

Congress in December 2010 and signed into law by President Obama in January 2011, requiring the development of a national strategic plan in order to address efforts to understanding and stopping the advance of Alzheimer's disease across the federal government.[93] The NIA plays a critical role in NAPA's objective of effectively treating or preventing Alzheimer's by 2025.

President Barack Obama has become increasingly aware of the pervasiveness of Alzheimer's disease. In his second term as President, he allocated an unprecedented $122 million for research, education, outreach, and caregiver support.[94] Although this amount of money is inconsequential when taking into account the national burden of Alzheimer's disease, it certainly is an adequate start towards ensuring that Alzheimer's research is properly funded and supported on a national scale. As part of the National Plan to Address Alzheimer's Disease, President Obama wanted to fuel the existing state of research aimed at uncovering the mysteries of the disease process and trying to find ways of modifying the destructive tendencies of the disease. The development of a national plan to address Alzheimer's disease is a critical step in the fight against the disease. However, much more must be done in order to effectively treat and manage this devastating medical condition. Interestingly, since the discovery of Alzheimer's disease in the early 20th century, very little has changed with regards to the outcomes of patients who develop the disease. The next chapter will explore the history of Alzheimer's disease and its discovery, as well as the history of the treatments, diagnostic techniques, and clinical trials that have focused on Alzheimer's.

References

1. http://www.alz.org/alzheimers_disease_early_onset.asp
2. Faden AI, Loane DJ. (2015) Chronic neurodegeneration after traumatic brain injury: Alzheimer disease, chronic traumatic encephalopathy, or persistent neuroinflammation? *Neurotherapeutics* **12**(1): 143–150.

3. Payami H, Zareparsi S, Montee KR, *et al.* (1996) Gender difference in apolipoprotein E-associated risk for familial Alzheimer disease: A possible clue to the higher incidence of Alzheimer disease in women. *Am J Hum Genet* **58**(4): 803–811.

4. http://www.ncbi.nlm.nih.gov/pmc/articles/PMC3891487/

5. Giedd JN, Raznahan A, Mills KL, *et al.* (2012) Review: Magnetic resonance imaging of male/female differences in human adolescent brain anatomy. *Biol Sex Differ* **3**(1): 19.

6. Cosgrove KP, Mazure CM, Staley JK. (2007) Evolving knowledge of sex differences in brain structure, function, and chemistry. *Biol Psychiatry* **62**(8): 847–855.

7. Perneczky R, Diehl-Schmid J, Förstl H, *et al.* (2007) Male gender is associated with greater cerebral hypometabolism in frontotemporal dementia: Evidence for sex-related cognitive reserve. *Int J Geriatr Psychiatry* **22**(11): 1135–1140.

8. Perneczky R, Drzezga A, Diehl-Schmid J, *et al.* (2007) Gender differences in brain reserve: An ^{18}F-FDG PET study in Alzheimer's disease. *J Neurol* **254**(10): 1395–1400.

9. Buckner RL, Snyder AZ, Shannon BJ, *et al.* (2005) Molecular, structural, and functional characterization of Alzheimer's disease: Evidence for a relationship between default activity, amyloid, and memory. *J Neurosci* **25**(34): 7709–7717.

10. Farrer LA, Cupples LA, Haines JL, *et al.* (1997) Effects of age, sex, and ethnicity on the association between apolipoprotein E genotype and Alzheimer disease. A meta-analysis. APOE and Alzheimer Disease Meta Analysis Consortium. *JAMA* **278**(16): 1349–1356.

11. Payami H, Zareparsi S, Montee KR, *et al.* (1996) Gender difference in apolipoprotein E-associated risk for familial Alzheimer disease: A possible clue to the higher incidence of Alzheimer disease in women. *Am J Hum Genet* **58**(4): 803–811.

12. Fukumoto N, Fujii T, Combarros O, *et al.* (2010) Sexually dimorphic effect of the Val66Met polymorphism of BDNF on susceptibility to Alzheimer's disease: New data and meta-analysis. *Am J Med Genet B Neuropsychiatry Genet* **153B**(1): 235–242.

13. Zou F, Gopalraj RK, Lok J, *et al.* (2008) Sex-dependent association of a common low-density lipoprotein receptor polymorphism with RNA splicing efficiency in the brain and Alzheimer's disease. *Hum Mol Genet* **17**(7): 929–935.

14. Hamilton G, Proitsi P, Jehu L, *et al.* (2007) Candidate gene association study of insulin signaling genes and Alzheimer's disease: Evidence for SOS2, PCK1, and PPARgamma as susceptibility loci. *Am J Med Genet B Neuropsychiatry Genet* **144B**(4): 508–516.

15. Morrison JH, Brinton RD, Schmidt PJ, Gore AC. (2006) Estrogen, menopause, and the aging brain: How basic neuroscience can inform hormone therapy in women. *J Neurosci.* **26**(41): 10332–10348.

16. Feldman HA, Longcope C, Derby CA, *et al.* (2002) Age trends in the level of serum testosterone and other hormones in middle-aged men: Longitudinal results from the Massachusetts male aging study. *J Clin Endocrinol Metab* **87**(2): 589–598.

17. Murphy DD, Segal M. (1996) Regulation of dendritic spine density in cultured rat hippocampal neurons by steroid hormones. *J Neurosci* **16**(13): 4059–4068.

18. Aenlle KK, Kumar A, Cui L, *et al.* (2009) Estrogen effects on cognition and hippocampal transcription in middle-aged mice. *Neurobiol Aging* **30**(6): 932–945.

19. Han X, Aenlle KK, Bean LA, *et al.* (2013) Role of estrogen receptor α and β in preserving hippocampal function during aging. *J Neurosci* **33**(6): 2671–2683.

20. Wang Q, Santizo R, Baughman VL, *et al.* (1999) Estrogen provides neuroprotection in transient forebrain ischemia through perfusion-independent mechanisms in rats. *Stroke* **30**(3): 630–637.

21. Gibbs RB. (1994) Estrogen and nerve growth factor-related systems in brain. Effects on basal forebrain cholinergic neurons and implications for learning and memory processes and aging. *Ann N Y Acad Sci* **743**: 165–196; discussion 197–199.

22. Gibbs RB, Aggarwal P. (1998) Estrogen and basal forebrain cholinergic neurons: Implications for brain aging and Alzheimer's disease-related cognitive decline. *Horm Behav* **34**(2): 98–111.

23. Nilsen J, Chen S, Irwin RW, *et al.* (2006) Estrogen protects neuronal cells from amyloid beta-induced apoptosis via regulation of mitochondrial proteins and function. *BMC Neurosci* **7**: 74.

24. Waring SC, Rocca WA, Petersen RC, *et al.* (1999) Postmenopausal estrogen replacement therapy and risk of AD: A population-based study. *Neurology* **52**(5): 965–970.

25. LeBlanc ES, Janowsky J, Chan BK, Nelson HD. (2001) Hormone replacement therapy and cognition: Systematic review and meta-analysis. *JAMA* **285**(11): 1489–1499.

26. Zandi PP, Carlson MC, Plassman BL, *et al.*; Cache County Memory Study Investigators. (2002) Hormone replacement therapy and incidence of Alzheimer disease in older women: The Cache County Study. *JAMA* **288**(17): 2123–2129.

27. Henderson VW, Benke KS, Green RC, *et al.*; MIRAGE Study Group. (2005) Postmenopausal hormone therapy and Alzheimer's disease risk: Interaction with age. *J Neurol Neurosurg Psychiatry* **76**(1): 103–105.

28. Whitmer RA, Quesenberry CP, Zhou J, Yaffe K. (2011) Timing of hormone therapy and dementia: The critical window theory revisited. *Ann Neurol* **69**(1): 163–169.

29. Rocca WA, Bower JH, Maraganore DM, *et al.* (2007) Increased risk of cognitive impairment or dementia in women who underwent oophorectomy before menopause. *Neurology* **69**(11): 1074–1083.

30. Shumaker SA, Legault C, Kuller L, *et al.* (2004) Conjugated equine estrogens and incidence of probable dementia and mild cognitive impairment in postmenopausal women: Women's Health Initiative Memory Study. *JAMA* **291**(24): 2947–2958.

31. Rocca WA, Grossardt BR, Shuster LT. (2010) Oophorectomy, menopause, estrogen, and cognitive aging: The timing hypothesis. *Neurodegener Dis* **7**(1–3): 163–166.

32. Zhang QG, Han D, Wang RM, *et al.* (2011) C terminus of Hsc70-interacting protein (CHIP)-mediated degradation of hippocampal estrogen receptor-alpha and the critical period hypothesis of estrogen neuroprotection. *Proc Natl Acad Sci USA* **108**(35): E617–E624.

33. Brinton RD. (2008) The healthy cell bias of estrogen action: Mitochondrial bioenergetics and neurological implications. *Trends Neurosci* **31**(10): 529–537.

34. Vemuri P, Lesnick TG, Przybelski SA, *et al.* (2012) Effect of lifestyle activities on Alzheimer disease biomarkers and cognition. *Ann Neurol* **72**(5): 730–738.

35. Katzman R. (1993) Education and the prevalence of dementia and Alzheimer's disease. *Neurology* **43**(1): 13–20.

36. Fratiglioni L, Grut M, Forsell Y, *et al.* (1991) Prevalence of Alzheimer's disease and other dementias in an elderly urban population: Relationship with age, sex, and education. *Neurology* **41**(12): 1886–1892.

37. Zhang MY, Katzman R, Salmon D, *et al.* (1990) The prevalence of dementia and Alzheimer's disease in Shanghai, China: Impact of age, gender, and education. *Ann Neurol* **27**(4): 428–437.

38. Bonaiuto S, Rocca WA, Lippi A, *et al.* (1995) Education and occupation as risk factors for dementia: A population-based case-control study. *Neuroepidemiology* **14**(3): 101–109.

39. Mortimer JA, Graves AB. (1993) Education and other socioeconomic determinants of dementia and Alzheimer's disease. *Neurology* **43**(8 Suppl. 4): S39–S44.

40. Karp A, Kåreholt I, Qiu C, *et al.* (2004) Relation of education and occupation-based socioeconomic status to incident Alzheimer's disease. *Am J Epidemiol* **159**(2): 175–183.

41. Bickel H, Cooper B. (1994) Incidence and relative risk of dementia in an urban elderly population: Findings of a prospective field study. *Psychol Med* **24**(1): 179–192.

42. Stern Y, Gurland B, Tatemichi TK, *et al.* (1994) Influence of education and occupation on the incidence of Alzheimer's disease. *JAMA* **271**(13): 1004–1010.

43. Roe CM, Xiong C, Miller JP, Morris JC. (2007) Education and Alzheimer disease without dementia: Support for the cognitive reserve hypothesis. *Neurology* **68**(3): 223–228.

44. Crowe M, Andel R, Pedersen NL, *et al.* (2003) Does participation in leisure activities lead to reduced risk of Alzheimer's disease? A prospective study of Swedish twins. *J Gerontol B Psychol Sci Soc Sci* **58**(5): P249–P255.

45. Fabrigoule C. (2002) Do leisure activities protect against Alzheimer's disease? *Lancet Neurol* **1**(1): 11.

46. Gale CR, Cooper R, Craig L, *et al.* (2012) Cognitive function in childhood and lifetime cognitive change in relation to mental wellbeing in four cohorts of older people. *PLoS One* **7**(9): e44860.

47. Whalley LJ, Starr JM, Athawes R, *et al.* (2000) Childhood mental ability and dementia. *Neurology* **55**(10): 1455–1459.

48. Whalley LJ, Deary IJ. (2001) Longitudinal cohort study of childhood IQ and survival up to age 76. *BMJ* **322**(7290): 819.

49. Scarmeas N, Zarahn E, Anderson KE, *et al.* (2003) Association of life activities with cerebral blood flow in Alzheimer disease: Implications for the cognitive reserve hypothesis. *Arch Neurol* **60**(3): 359–365.

50. Garibotto V, Borroni B, Kalbe E, *et al.* (2008) Education and occupation as proxies for reserve in aMCI converters and AD: FDG-PET evidence. *Neurology* **71**(17): 1342–1349.

51. Kemppainen NM, Aalto S, Karrasch M, *et al.* (2008) Cognitive reserve hypothesis: Pittsburgh compound B and fluorodeoxyglucose positron emission tomography in relation to education in mild Alzheimer's disease. *Ann Neurol* **63**(1): 112–118.

52. Roe CM, Mintun MA, D'Angelo G, *et al.* (2008) Alzheimer disease and cognitive reserve: Variation of education effect with carbon 11-labeled Pittsburgh compound B uptake. *Arch Neurol* **65**(11): 1467–1471.

53. Schneider AL, Sharrett AR, Patel MD, *et al.* (2012) Education and cognitive change over 15 years: The Atherosclerosis Risk in Communities Study. *J Am Geriatr Soc* **60**(10): 1847–1853.

54. Geda YE, Roberts RO, Knopman DS, *et al.* (2010) Physical exercise, aging, and mild cognitive impairment: A population-based study. *Arch Neurol* **67**(1): 80–86.

55. Hamer M, Chida Y. (2009) Physical activity and risk of neurodegenerative disease: A systematic review of prospective evidence. *Psychol Med* **39**(1): 3–11.

56. Middleton LE, Barnes DE, Lui LY, Yaffe K. (2010) Physical activity over the life course and its association with cognitive performance and impairment in old age. *J Am Geriatr Soc* **58**(7): 1322–1326.

57. Liu R, Sui X, Laditka JN, *et al.* (2012) Cardiorespiratory fitness as a predictor of dementia mortality in men and women. *Med Sci Sports Exerc* **44**(2): 253–259.

58. Buchman AS, Boyle PA, Yu L, *et al.* (2012) Total daily physical activity and the risk of AD and cognitive decline in older adults. *Neurology* **78**(17): 1323–1329.

59. Geda YE, Roberts RO, Knopman DS, *et al.* (2010) Physical exercise, aging, and mild cognitive impairment: A population-based study. *Arch Neurol* **67**(1): 80–86.

60. Nomaguchi KM, Bianchi SM. (2004) Exercise time: Gender differences in the effects of marriage, parenthood, and employment. *J Marriage Fam* **66**(2): 413–430.

61. Hogervorst E, Clifford A, Stock J, *et al.* (2012) Exercise to prevent cognitive decline and Alzheimer's disease: For whom, when, what, and (most importantly) how much? *J Alzheimers Dis Park* **2**(3): e117.

62. Clifford A, Bandelow S, Hogervorst E. (2010) The effects of physical exercise on cognitive function in the elderly: A review. In: Gariépy Q, Ménard R (eds). *Handbook of Cognitive Aging: Causes, Processes and Effects*. New York, NY: Nova Science Publishers. pp. 109–150.

63. Fallah N, Mitnitski A, Middleton L, Rockwood K. (2009) Modeling the impact of sex on how exercise is associated with cognitive changes and death in older Canadians. *Neuroepidemiology* **33**(1): 47–54.

64. http://www.cdc.gov/mmwr/preview/mmwrhtml/mm6347a4.htm?s_cid=mm6347a4_w

65. Launer LJ, Andersen K, Dewey ME, *et al.* (1999) Rates and risk factors for dementia and Alzheimer's disease: Results from EURODEM pooled analyses. EURODEM Incidence Research Group and Work Groups. European Studies of Dementia. *Neurology* **52**(1): 78–84.

66. Rezvani AH, Levin ED. (2001) Cognitive effects of nicotine. *Biol Psychiatry* **49**(3): 258–267.

67. Wilson AL, Langley LK, Monley J, *et al.* (1995) Nicotine patches in Alzheimer's disease: Pilot study on learning, memory, and safety. *Pharmacol Biochem Behav* **51**(2–3): 509–514.

68. White HK, Levin ED. (1999) Four-week nicotine skin patch treatment effects on cognitive performance in Alzheimer's disease. *Psychopharmacology (Berl)* **143**(2): 158–165.

69. Hagger-Johnson G, Sabia S, Brunner EJ, *et al.* (2013) Combined impact of smoking and heavy alcohol use on cognitive decline in early old age: Whitehall II prospective cohort study. *Br J Psychiatry* **203**(2): 120–125.

70. Moreno-Gonzalez I, Estrada LD, Sanchez-Mejias E, Soto C. (2013) Smoking exacerbates amyloid pathology in a mouse model of Alzheimer's disease. *Nat Commun* 4: 1495.

71. Ho YS, Yang X, Yeung SC, *et al.* (2012) Cigarette smoking accelerated brain aging and induced pre-Alzheimer-like neuropathology in rats. *PLoS One* **7**(5): e36752.

72. Ott A, Slooter AJ, Hofman A, *et al.* (1998) Smoking and risk of dementia and Alzheimer's disease in a population-based cohort study: The Rotterdam Study. *Lancet* **351**(9119): 1840–1843.

73. Rusanen M, Kivipelto M, Quesenberry CP Jr, *et al.* (2011) Heavy smoking in midlife and long-term risk of Alzheimer disease and vascular dementia. *Arch Intern Med* **171**(4): 333–339.

74. Tyas SL, White LR, Petrovitch H, *et al.* (2003) Mid-life smoking and late-life dementia: The Honolulu–Asia Aging Study. *Neurobiol Aging* **24**(4): 589–596.

75. Durazzo TC, Insel PS, Weiner MW; Alzheimer Disease Neuroimaging Initiative. (2012) Greater regional brain atrophy rate in healthy elderly subjects with a history of cigarette smoking. *Alzheimers Dement* **8**(6): 513–519.

76. Barnes LL, Bennett DA. (2014) Alzheimer's disease in African Americans: Risk factors and challenges for the future. *Health Affairs* **33**(4): 580–586.

77. https://www.alz.co.uk/research/WorldAlzheimerReport2015.pdf

78. http://www.alzheimersanddementia.com/article/S1552-5260(12)02531-9/abstract

79. http://www.alz.org/facts/downloads/facts_figures_2015.pdf

80. Prince M, Albanese E, Guerchet M, Prina M. (2014) *World Alzheimer Report 2014. Dementia and Risk Reduction. An analysis of Protective and Modifiable Risk Factors*. London: Alzheimer's Disease International.

81. Chan KY, Wang W, Wu JJ, *et al.* (2013) Epidemiology of Alzheimer's disease and other forms of dementia in China, 1990–2010: A systematic review and analysis. *Lancet* **381**(9882): 2016–2023.

82. http://www.alz.co.uk/research/GlobalImpactDementia2013.pdf

83. http://www.alz.co.uk/research/G8-policy-brief

84. https://www.nia.nih.gov/research/dn/international-alzheimers-disease-research-portfolio

85. http://report.nih.gov/categorical_spending.aspx

86. http://www.nih.gov/about-nih/what-we-do/budget

87. http://report.nih.gov/categorical_spending.aspx

88. https://www.alz.org/documents_custom/trajectory.pdf

89. http://www.foodallergy.org/document.doc?id=46

90. http://www.alz.org/documents/national/submitted-testimony-050113.pdf

91. http://en.wikipedia.org/wiki/National_Institute_on_Aging

92. https://www.nia.nih.gov/about/nia-timeline

93. http://napa.alz.org/national-alzheimers-project-act-background

94. http://www.alz.org/news_and_events_law_by_Obama.asp

7 The History of Alzheimer's Disease

"Those who do not remember the past are condemned to repeat it."
— George Santayana, philosopher, poet, novelist

The Characterization of the Disease by Dr. Alzheimer in the Early 1900s

"Alzheimer's disease" is sometimes mistaken by individuals as "old-timers' disease." This term even makes some sense, because it was almost always associated with senior citizens. Well, individuals with this misconception soon figure out that there is no such thing as old-timers' disease; rather, Alzheimer's disease is the culprit.

The story of the discovery of Alzheimer's disease begins on June 14, 1864, when Aloysius "Alois" Alzheimer was born in a small town known as Marktbriet in Southern Germany. Alois had a knack for science, and grew up to study medicine, graduating from the universities of Aschaffenburg, Tubingen, Berlin, and Würsburg as a doctor in 1887 (Fig. 7.1). After graduating, Alois completed a residency in psychiatry and neuropathology in Frankfurt, Germany, at an institution known as the "Hospital for the Mentally Ill and Epileptics."[1] This hospital was run by Emil Sioli, a well-known psychiatrist, and employed Franz Nissl, a famous neuropathologist. Alois worked closely with these two individuals and eventually came to study nervous system pathology. In collaboration with Franz Nissl, Alois Alzheimer helped publish a six-volume series entitled *Histologic and Histopathologic Studies of the Cerebral Cortex*

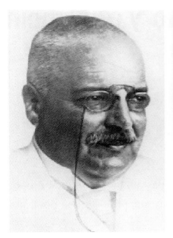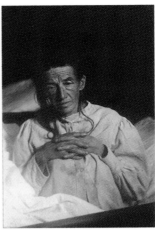

Fig. 7.1. Dr. Alois Alzheimer (left) and Auguste Deter (right). Pictured here in 1901, Deter was Dr. Alois Alzheimer's patient and the first patient to be described with Alzheimer's disease. (Figure credits: Refs. 2 and 3.)

from 1907 to 1918. Prior to the publication of his volume, Alois began working with Emil Kraepelin, a well-known German psychiatrist at the Munich School of Medicine in 1903.

Alois continued to study the brain and its disorders, and in 1906, Dr. Alois Alzheimer gave a famous lecture in which he described various cognitive changes that he had observed in a patient of his. This patient was a 51-year-old woman named Auguste Deter, who was deemed to be delusional and psychotic, and was admitted to an asylum in Frankfurt in 1901. The patient exhibited very odd behavioral problems including a profound loss of short-term memory. At the time, Deter's case sparked interest in Dr. Alzheimer and she became the focal point of his research. To his advantage, he was able to strike a deal in order to receive her records and brain upon her death in order to continue his work.

On autopsy, Dr. Alzheimer recognized a profound decrease in the overall size and mass of Deter's brain, clinically known as atrophy. Along with the dramatic decrease in size, Dr. Alzheimer noted abnormal deposits within and around the brain cells. As a well-known psychiatrist and neuropathologist, he presented the first documented case of the disease on November 4, 1906, at a medical conference in Germany. After Dr. Alzheimer made these discoveries, a German colleague of his, Dr. Emil Kraepelin, coined the term "Alzheimer's disease" in reference to Dr. Alzheimer's patient in the eighth edition of his book, *Psychiatrie*. Although the condition was not referred to as Alzheimer's disease until 1915, by 1911, the description of the disease was being used by European physicians to diagnose patients in the United States. Unfortunately, in 1913, Alois fell ill to an infection and developed rheumatic fever and endocarditis (an inflammation of the inner lining of the heart). This illness led to Alois' death in 1915 at 51 years of age, and later he was buried in Wroclaw, Poland, next to his wife.

As scientific progress continued, the nature of the abnormal deposits that Dr. Alois Alzheimer had initially described were elucidated. With the advent of the electron microscope in 1931 and the further study of Alzheimer's disease, scientists discovered that the abnormal deposits were composed of abnormally modified proteins. These proteins are known as β-amyloid and tau. β-amyloid is a major component of the plaques that are classically found *outside* of the neurons and disrupt the connections between neurons. Conversely, tau is a key component of tangles, which are found *within* the neurons and disrupt the transmission of signals. Thus, the hallmark histological (microscopic) features of Alzheimer's disease are plaques and tangles.

Interestingly, although the elucidation of the plaques and tangles was achieved in the mid-1980s, the relationship between the plaques and tangles and Alzheimer's disease remains unclear. It is still unknown whether or not the plaques and tangles cause the disease or if they are a result of the disease process itself. The notion that the plaques and tangles are in fact byproducts of a chronically ongoing disease process and represent the later or end stage of the Alzheimer's process is becoming increasingly accepted. Recently, there has been an increased focus on the overall "health" of the neurons and the environment in which they are found, and less of an emphasis on the abnormal proteins that are present. Furthermore, the focus has shifted beyond the individual neuron and onto glial cells, biomarkers, lymphatics, and other parts of the brain. Nonetheless, plaques and tangles are important hallmarks of Alzheimer's disease. This finding has driven many scientists to try to understand what role these key elements play in the disease process and how changing the make-up of the plaques and tangles can modify the disease. Several drugs have been formulated that seek to diminish the plaque load within the brain, and it has been indicated that doing so could improve cognitive outcomes in Alzheimer's patients; however, a 2008 clinical trial in which a vaccine that generated an immune response against plaques unfortunately lead to a severe life-threatening complication known as meningoencephalitis. Because of this, the clinical trial had to be stopped and the drug was reformulated with the hopes that the deadly side effect could be avoided in future trials.[4,5]

This early vaccine was known as AN1792, and it effectively activated the body's immune system to fight against the β-amyloid protein fragments that form the plaques in Alzheimer's disease.[6,7] However, since 6% of the individuals who received AN1792 developed meningoencephalitis, which is a severe inflammation of the brain and the meninges, the trial was immediately stopped. The reason for the severe side effect of AN1792 is that the white blood cells that were supposed to attack the β-amyloid plaques ended up instead attacking normal brain tissue.

The reformulated vaccine, known as CAD106, was given to 58 individuals with mild-to-moderate Alzheimer's disease in 2012. The majority — approximately 75% — of individuals who received CAD106 developed antibodies against the β-amyloid protein, a sign of effectiveness. Although none of the 58 individuals developed meningoencephalitis since CAD106 targets only β-amyloid protein, they did report several side effects, including airway inflammation, headache, muscle pain, and fatigue.

Recently, in 2015, the results of the long-term use of CAD106 were reported. Fortunately, the preliminary results showed no unexpected side effects or safety findings and an absence of a β-amyloid-specific immune cell response. This supports the CAD106 "favorable tolerability profile," meaning that so far, it seems to be safe and well tolerated by patients who received it.[8] These results indicate that the CAD106 vaccine may prove to be an effective treatment in Alzheimer's disease by alleviating the plaque burden in patients. However, decreasing the plaque burden alone may not be enough to treat or cure Alzheimer's disease, and a combinatorial approach to treatment that includes ameliorating the formation of the neurofibrillary tangles may be needed.

The Development of the Diagnostic Tools

An interesting analogy between Alzheimer's disease and heart (cardiovascular) disease can be made. Cardiovascular disease is very prevalent, just like Alzheimer's disease, and it is a slow-growing and devastating disease that kills millions of people worldwide each year. But cardiovascular disease has very well-defined risk factors and biomarkers, with a simple blood test being able to examine cholesterol, glucose, fat, and much more. This simple blood panel provides physicians with a plethora of information on that patient's likelihood of progressing onto cardiovascular disease, and allows preventative measures to be taken prior to the onset of symptoms. However, Alzheimer's disease has not classically had any well-determined and efficacious biological markers that allowed physicians to accurately predict the risk of developing Alzheimer's. An increasingly substantial scientific shift that is focusing on identifying biomarkers for Alzheimer's disease has been underway. From blood tests, cerebrospinal fluid studies, brain imaging, neurological, and psychological examinations, and more, the development of biomarkers has become an increasingly critical component in the war against Alzheimer's disease. The classical "markers" and tests that have allowed physicians to predict the trajectory of an individual presenting with memory changes that are indicative of dementia have been primarily neuropsychological examinations, history taking, and a neurological examination (to rule out other disorders from the differential diagnosis).

Additionally, blood work and brain scans can help rule out other possible disorders, but do not provide a definitive diagnosis. Neuropsychological examinations are batteries of tests that evaluate mental functioning. They are cognitive and subjective in nature, and thus less tangible than "hard" biomarkers such as cholesterol.

Currently, the best way to treat cardiovascular disease is to prevent it. This same approach holds true for nearly any disease, including Alzheimer's. If a disease can be prevented from occurring or can have its course modified, the trajectory of a patient's life can be altered. The problem has been figuring out how to catch the disease early on and how to modify its course. The development of rigorous neuropsychiatric questionnaires and assessments have led to the creation of "cognitive" profiles of individuals at various stages of cognitive decline. By administering a pre-determined battery of questions, puzzles, and tasks to patients who are being evaluated for dementia, the results can assist neurologists in determining who is at risk of the development of Alzheimer's disease and who is not. This is in combination with a thorough family history, medical history, and neurological examination. The success of using cognitive performance as an index of disease progression has allowed physicians to identify mild cognitive difficulties up to 8 years before an individual fulfills the clinical criteria for Alzheimer's disease.

However, even the best methods of early diagnosis are insufficient. According to Eric Greb, the Senior Associate Editor of *Neurology Reviews*, "Because of a lack of effective clinical tools, neurologists can only diagnose Alzheimer's disease definitively through a neuropathologic examination at autopsy. The sensitivity and specificity of clinical diagnoses of Alzheimer's disease vary according to the neuropathologic criteria used, and false positives may account for 12% to 23% of patients diagnosed with Alzheimer's disease."[9] False positives mean that up to a quarter of patients are misdiagnosed as having Alzheimer's disease, when in reality they did not have it, based on autopsy findings.

In addition, it is very difficult to predict which individuals will develop Alzheimer's disease and which will not. What really is needed is a biomarker — just like cholesterol for heart disease — that allows physicians to stratify patients according to their risk of progressing onto Alzheimer's disease, and would allow for early prophylactic (preventative) treatment of those patients. Another reason that early diagnosis and biomarkers are important is that a biomarker that can detect the earliest signs of Alzheimer's disease can allow scientists to conduct clinical tests using new treatments on patients before those patients develop Alzheimer's disease. For example, patients in their late 50s could be enrolled in a long-term study that would monitor their blood for a biomarker that is specific to Alzheimer's disease. Some of those patients could then be placed on a new experimental treatment regimen, while the others would receive standard or no treatment. The patients would then be followed for 5–10 years, and the percentages of patients who develop Alzheimer's disease in each group could be determined. If the group receiving the treatment develops Alzheimer's disease to a lesser degree than the untreated group, then it is possible that the treatment worked. Additionally, the use of biomarkers throughout the course of the study would allow the researchers to better understand what levels of the particular biomarker correlate with the onset of Alzheimer's disease. If this is determined, then once a treatment emerges in the future, individuals who are at a high risk of developing Alzheimer's disease based on their biomarker analysis could be placed on disease-altering medications well before the onset of clinical symptoms. There will be more on this topic later.

The Development of Medications

In 1987, the world's first Alzheimer's drug trial got underway. This drug, tacrine (Cognex), became approved for human use by the Food and Drug Administration (FDA) in 1993. Over the next 10 years, four more drugs became available. This was an apparent victory for patients and physicians in the fight against Alzheimer's disease. Unfortunately, due to the inability of these drugs to cure Alzheimer's disease or drastically modify its course, the triumph was fleeting.

Table 7.1. Food and Drug Administration-Approved Medications for Alzheimer's Disease

Medication	Brand name	FDA approval year	Approval For
Donepezil	Aricept	1996	All stages
Rivastigmine	Exelon	2000	All stages
Galantamine	Razadyne	2001	Mild to moderate
Memantine	Namenda	2003	Moderate to severe
Tacrine (donepezil and memantine)	Cognex	1993	Mild to moderate

There are currently five drugs that are FDA approved in the USA for the treatment of Alzheimer's disease — none cure the disease (Table 7.1). These include cholinesterase inhibitors (CHIs; donepezil, rivastigmine, and galantamine), an N-methyl-d-aspartate (NMDA) channel blocker (memantine), or a combination of both mechanisms (donepezil and memantine).

Acetylcholine is an important neurotransmitter that is involved in memory and Alzheimer's disease. The pathways that produce and distribute acetylcholine — known as cholinergic pathways — in the cerebral cortex and basal forebrain are compromised in Alzheimer's disease. This deficit is thought to contribute to the cognitive impairment we see in the disease.[10] Acetylcholine is broken down by a protein known as acetylcholinesterase, or cholinesterase for short. Thus, a class of drugs known as CHIs is given in order to prevent the further breakdown of acetylcholine. CHIs have been clinically shown to delay the worsening of symptoms for approximately 6–12 months in about half of the individuals who take them. Donepezil is approved for the treatment of all stages of Alzheimer's, while rivastigmine and galantamine are approved for the treatment of mild-to-moderate Alzheimer's disease primarily.[11]

In the brain, a different neurotransmitter that is involved in the activation or "excitation" of neurons, known as glutamate, is also involved in learning and memory. Glutamate binds to a particular protein known as an NMDA receptor and plays an important role in synaptic plasticity, normal memory, and learning new tasks. In Alzheimer's disease, excess glutamate can be released from damaged cells, resulting in large amounts of calcium entering the cell. Chronic overexposure to calcium can lead to cell damage and death. This process is known as glutamatergic excitotoxicity (toxicity to the cell that is mediated by the excitatory neurotransmitter glutamate). Memantine helps prevent this destructive chain of events by partially blocking the NMDA receptors. Memantine generally modified the progressive symptomatic decline in global status, cognition, function, and behavior of patients with moderate-to-severe Alzheimer's disease in four 12- to 28-week clinical trials. In patients with mild-to-moderate Alzheimer's disease, the data from three 24-week trials are inconclusive, although some analyses show positive effects on global status and cognition.[12]

A combination of CHIs and NMDA receptor blockers is used for patients with moderate-to-severe Alzheimer's disease. The DOMINO-AD study was a 15-center, double-blind, randomized controlled trial at King's College London. The 2-year (2009–2011) study tested the efficacy of donepezil, memantine, and combination therapy in moderate-to-severe Alzheimer's disease patients.[13] The study noted that the best cognitive outcome was observed for patients taking donepezil alone, who showed approximately 32% less cognitive decline than those on placebo. There were positive cognitive outcomes for taking only memantine, but to a lesser extent, with approximately 20% less decline than those on placebo. Unfortunately, the study concluded that combined treatment with both donepezil and memantine was not better than treatment with donepezil alone for any of the trial's measured outcomes.[14]

As cognitive-enhancing drugs, the five FDA-approved drug therapies demonstrate only mild-to-moderate effects on memory and activities of daily living, inducing a delay of progression for approximately 6–12 months, with stable efficacy over years.[15] In addition to these, there are drugs that address the non-cognitive complications of Alzheimer's disease, such as depression. These include antipsychotics, antidepressants, and benzodiazepines medications. Unfortunately, these pharmacological agents have shown limited efficacy and poor safety outcomes in randomized controlled trials. The adverse events that come with atypical antipsychotics lead to an increased risk of dropouts.[16]

To sum up, the drugs described above have proven to be safe and clinically efficacious in the treatment of Alzheimer's disease. However, they do not significantly alter the course of the disease. Patients who are afflicted with the disease and are started on these drugs continue to deteriorate. It is unfortunate and confusing that these drugs, which held such promise, had such few tangible benefits to patients and their families.

One of the hopes when starting patients on anti-Alzheimer's medications is to slow the progression of the disease process and improve cognitive capacity in the interim. The various drugs that were FDA approved for this purpose simply do not do enough. An analogy would be trying to stop a plane from crashing, but giving it an extra 30 seconds of flight before it crashed — the drugs simply do not do enough. They do not significantly alter the disease trajectory nor stop the progression of the disease. They slightly enhance cognitive capacity on a certain set of neuropsychological tests that are commonly used in the assessment and follow-up of patients with Alzheimer's disease. These slight drug-related improvements were orders of magnitude below what would be considered a cure, but just significant enough to warrant their use given the side-effect profiles of the drugs. Nonetheless, these drugs are the best weapons in our current arsenal, and they should be used along with lifestyle modifications and early diagnosis until better therapeutics emerge.

In addition to efficacy, cost-effectiveness has been studied and will be increasingly scrutinized as cost-containment of healthcare becomes a higher priority. The average cost per patient for one of these drugs is non-trivial. In the USA, the drugs cost $5 per day on average, or approximately $1,800 annually per patient.[17]

Currently, Medicare will cover generic forms of Alzheimer's drugs, but not the brand name versions (i.e. all forms of Aricept are no longer covered). Most plans have also imposed quantity limits (QLs) on the drugs.[18] In 2005, the British National Health Service (NHS), acting on guidance from the British National Institute for Health and Care Excellence (NICE), proposed to end the availability of CHIs and memantine for most of England's patients with Alzheimer's disease due to questions regarding cost-effectiveness.[19] This led to an outcry from patient, advocacy, and pharmaceutical groups that was loud enough for the UK organization to amend its policies two times in 4 years. As of 2009, NICE recommends CHIs for managing mild-to-moderate Alzheimer's disease, and memantine for people who cannot take CHIs and as an option for managing severe Alzheimer's disease.[20]

Clinical Trials Overview

Modern medicine is continually evolving and making rapid advances. In spite of the plethora of knowledge in relation to certain diseases and available drugs, there are some conditions that leave us helpless with unanswered questions. In order to overcome the challenges of well-known and newly discovered diseases, it is crucial to develop medications that will prolong a patient's life or eradicate a particular disease. The best way to defeat a disease or learn more about a certain type of drug or vaccine is to perform a series of clinical studies. A clinical trial is medical research that delves into the treatments, strategies, and devices used to combat a disease in order to test the safety and effectiveness of each. These substances and devices are then tested in humans, in something known as a clinical trial.

In clinical trials, patient safety is the most important consideration. Additionally, all clinical trials must be conducted in accordance with specific rules and requirements in order to protect the patients' rights and to keep them safe during the study. These trials are held in research institutions or specialized hospitals in order to meet specific guidelines. All new medications and devices are checked in order to ensure that the materials used are harmless and will guarantee safety. Individuals of all ages can voluntarily participate in clinical trials or they can be recommended to participate by their physicians. In order to test the effectiveness of a specific treatment, the voluntary subjects participating in the trials can be either healthy or sick. Clinical trials provide useful information on the safety and efficacy of a new medical therapy and shed light on any associated risks.

Clinical trials are split into five phases (see Table 7.2). Each phase is unique and provides different results in order to provide answers to the specific question being studied. Once a positive result has been obtained, the researchers move on to the next stage of the clinical trial. Prior to the beginning of Phase I, a pre-clinical phase called Phase 0 is conducted. The pre-clinical studies are not performed on humans; instead, they are conducted using test tubes, cell cultures, and animals. Such studies will allow researchers to proceed with the development of the new drug once the scientific and ethical boundaries have been met.

In Phase I, researchers begin to test the new drug or treatment in a small number of people in order to ensure that the drug is safe and can continue to be tested in subsequent phases. The drug's metabolism, toxicity, excretion, absorption, and possible interactions with other medications or substances such as food are examined. This phase is critical because not only is the drug's safety evaluated, but also the dosage range and side effects are determined.

Upon completion of Phase I, the drug is then administered to a larger group. This is Phase II of the clinical trial, in which a larger number of participants is given the drug in order to further evaluate the drug's (or treatment's) safety and potency. A detailed assessment in Phase II includes information regarding the absorption, metabolism, and excretion of the drug, depending on the patient's gender and age. Additionally, the drug is compared to commonly used treatments and placebo. The placebo is a control variable that is used when testing new drugs and it has no therapeutic effects on the patient. Additionally, this phase is "double-blinded," which means that neither the patient nor the researcher know whether the patient is given the test medication or placebo.

Table 7.2.   Clinical Trial Phases[21]

Phase	Purpose	Dose	Number of subjects	Notes
Preclinical	Testing and evaluation in non-human subjects	Variable	Not applicable	—
0	Evaluation of safety in a small number of human subjects	Sub-therapeutic	10–15	Sometimes skipped
I	Evaluation of dosage in healthy human subjects	Sub-therapeutic to therapeutic	20–100	Evaluates drug safety
II	Evaluation of safety and efficacy in human patients	Therapeutic	100–300	—
III	Evaluation of effectiveness, safety, and efficacy in human patients	Therapeutic	1000–2000	Evaluates therapeutic effect
IV	Post-marketing surveillance: evaluation of long-term success and impact on patients to find out more about the benefits or any side effects	Therapeutic		Evaluate long-term effects

Phase III aims to provide the drug or treatment to several hundred to several thousand patients, and can take several years to complete. Similarly to Phase II trials, Phase III trials involve randomizing which patients receive the test medication or placebo. Phase III allows pharmaceutical companies to gather large amounts of useful information on the new drug and ensure its safety. Following the completion of Phase III, a pharmaceutical company can request FDA approval in order to advertise and sell the drug.

The final stage of a clinical trial — Phase IV — involves ongoing surveillance of the drug in the mass market after the drug or treatment has been approved and widely sold. During this stage, the treatment is already marketed and used by patients around the United States and is readily available for purchase with a prescription. This final yet essential stage aims to determine whether the drug is safe for the general public and seeks to find rare side effects that went unnoticed during the first three phases of the clinical trial. During Phase IV trials, the drug's long-term success and impact on patients' lives is monitored. If necessary, these data would allow companies to place restrictions on the new drug and/or, in some cases, remove it from the market.

In the 1990s, scientists began working on experimental treatments that would theoretically cure Alzheimer's disease. Since the hallmark pathological features of Alzheimer's disease were plaques and tangles, it was thought that creating drugs that targeted these proteins would stop the disease process. One approach to this was the creation of vaccines. Two companies — Elan and Wyeth — created an experimental vaccine that would trick the body into bolstering an immune response against the tangles within the brain. This was successful in that it effectively reduced the tangle load within the brain; however, the clinical trial (which had entered Phase II) was stopped in 2002 when several patients who were taking the drug suffered deadly meningoencephalitis (basically, the brain and its protective coating became inflamed).

Over 1,500 clinical trials have gotten underway globally, aiming to determine how to alter the course of Alzheimer's disease. One of the reasons for the overwhelming failure of these trials is the ubiquitous nature of the disease. It does not affect just one part of the brain; rather, it affects the entire brain. This makes it extremely difficult to target. It is also difficult for drugs to enter the brain itself, due to an endogenous protective mechanism known as the blood–brain barrier (BBB), which is meant to prevent toxins from entering the brain. Unfortunately, this also prevents many drugs that may help treat Alzheimer's disease from entering the brain as well. The BBB can be thought of as a filter that prohibits many molecules, toxins, and proteins from entering into the brain. It is normally extremely important for protecting the brain from anything that could harm it. It does this by creating extremely tight junctions between the cells that make up the walls of the arteries within the brain. Normally, the junctions between these cells are leaky and allow fluid and other molecules to seep through, but in the brain, these cells are extremely tight and only let certain things through. Thus, in the development of drugs that are supposed to exert their effects on the brain, it is essential to formulate them with specific properties that allow them to pass through the BBB and into the brain.

Solanezumab

One large Phase III clinical trial is being conducted between 2014 and 2018 by a pharmaceutical company known as Eli Lilly. It is currently being conducted in 56 US sites, four Canadian sites, and one Australian site.[22,23] According to the National Institute on Aging (NIA), the anti-amyloid treatment in asymptomatic Alzheimer's disease (A4)study is testing the effects of a new drug known as solanezumab on slowing the progression of memory problems in Alzheimer's disease.[24] It is a Phase III clinical trial that is enrolling individuals between 65 and 85 years of age who have high levels of amyloid in the brain. Amyloid levels can be determined by a brain imaging technique known as positron emission tomography (PET). Specifically, a molecule known as Pittsburgh Compound B (PiB) or Amyvid is injected into a patient. This molecule is labeled with a radioactive tracer that courses through the bloodstream and can specifically bind to certain targeted proteins of interest. Both PiB and Amyvid bind to amyloid in the brain, and amyloid levels can be detected by the PET scanner. Patients with higher-than-normal levels of amyloid in the brain are therefore being enrolled in the A4 trial. These patients are then asked to receive either an intravenous infusion (IV) of solanezumab or a placebo every 4 weeks for 3 years. They are also asked to participate in memory tests and undergo electrocardiograms (ECG) to monitor cardiac function, brain scans (including PET scans), and blood tests.

Solanezumab is a drug that is classified as a "humanized monoclonal IgG1 antibody." Although this is a mouthful, is simply means that the drug is isolated and works in humans and specifically targets a protein. In the case of solanezumab, the protein that is targeted is β-amyloid. Specifically, the drug targets β-amyloid when it is in its soluble "monomer" form, meaning that it has not yet self-aggregated. It is thought that by binding to the single pieces of β-amyloid, solanezumab is able to prevent self-aggregation and the formation of plaques, which can harm neurons. In pre-clinical trials, solanezumab was able to reverse memory problems in mouse models of Alzheimer's disease. In Phase I studies in the USA and Japan, solanezumab was shown to be well-tolerated and had no major side effects. Phase II studies confirmed solanezumab's safety and tolerability, and also showed that the levels of β-amyloid in the CSF were elevated. Phase III studies called EXPEDITION-1 and -2 looked at 2,052 individuals with mild-to-moderate Alzheimer's disease, and although the safety of solanezumab was confirmed, it did not show significant effects in terms of reducing cognitive decline in Alzheimer's disease. However, there was a trend that appeared late in the study of mitigation of cognitive deterioration, suggesting that solanezumab may actually modify the Alzheimer's disease process. EXPEDITION-3 was started by Eli Lilly and enrolled 2,100 patients with mild Alzheimer's disease; however, the results have not yet been released (results are expected to be out in December 2016). Furthermore, solanezumab was chosen to be used in two other studies, with the Dominantly Inherited Alzheimer's Network (DIAN) and the Alzheimer's Disease Cooperative Study both using solanezumab in order to look at its effects on genetically inherited Alzheimer's disease, as well as its effects on patients with high levels of amyloid in the brain. This latter study is the A4 study, and is expected to be completed by 2020.

References

1. http://www.biography.com/people/alois-alzheimer-21216461
2. https://commons.wikimedia.org/wiki/File:Auguste_D_aus_Marktbreit.jpg
3. https://commons.wikimedia.org/wiki/File:Alois_Alzheimer_003.jpg
4. Wisniewski T, Konietzko U. (2008) Amyloid-β immunisation for Alzheimer's disease. *Lancet Neurol* **7**(9): 805–811.
5. Lambracht-Washington D, Rosenberg RN. (2013) Advances in the development of vaccines for Alzheimer's disease. *Discov Med* **15**(84): 319–326.
6. Vellas B, Black R, Thal LJ, *et al*. (2009) Long-term follow-up of patients immunized with AN1792: Reduced functional decline in antibody responders. *Curr Alzheimer Res* **6**(2): 144–151.
7. http://www.health.harvard.edu/blog/early-steps-toward-an-alzheimers-vaccine-201206124878
8. Farlow MR, Andreasen N, Riviere ME, *et al*. (2015) Long-term treatment with active Aβ immunotherapy with CAD106 in mild Alzheimer's disease. *Alzheimers Res Ther* **7**(1): 23.
9. http://www.neurologyreviews.com/the-publication/issue-single-view/misdiagnosis-of-alzheimers-disease-is-linked-to-less-severe-dementia-profile/d1c636cd06700c30110c41d1d0499110.html
10. Becker RE. (1991) Therapy of the cognitive deficit in Alzheimer's disease; the cholinergic system. In: Becker RE, Giacobini E (eds). *Cholinergic Basis of Alzheimer Therapy*. Boston, MA: Berkhauser, pp. 1–22.
11. http://www.alz.org/alzheimers_disease_standard_prescriptions.asp
12. Robinson DM, Keating GM. (2006) Memantine. *Drugs* **66**(11): 1515–1534.
13. Jones R, Sheehan B, Phillips P, *et al*.; DOMINO-AD team. (2009) DOMINO-AD protocol: Donepezil and memantine in moderate to severe Alzheimer's disease. *Trials* **10**: 57.

14. Howard R, McShane R, Lindesay J, *et al*. (2012) Donepezil and memantine for moderate-to-severe Alzheimer's disease. *N Engl J Med* **366**(10): 893–903.

15. http://emjreviews.com/therapeutic-area/neurology/update-on-alzheimers-disease/

16. Wang J, Yu JT, Wang HF, *et al*. (2015) Pharmacological treatment of neuropsychiatric symptoms in Alzheimer's disease: A systematic review and meta-analysis. *J Neurol Neurosurg Psychiatry* **86**: 101–109.

17. Casey DA, Antimisiaris D, O'Brien J. (2010) Drugs for Alzheimer's disease: Are they effective? *Pharm Ther* **35**(4): 208–211.

18. https://www.alz.org/care/alzheimers-dementia-medicare-part-d.asp

19. National Institute for Clinical Excellence (NICE). Alzheimer's disease: Donepezil, galantamine, rivastigmine (review) and memantine. [www.nice.org.uk/guidance/TA111].

20. http://www.nice.org.uk/guidance/ta217

21. https://en.wikipedia.org/wiki/Phases_of_clinical_research

22. https://www.clinicaltrials.gov/ct2/show/study/NCT02008357

23. https://www.nia.nih.gov/alzheimers/a4-study

24. https://www.nia.nih.gov/alzheimers/clinical-trials/anti-amyloid-treatment-asymptomatic-alzheimers-disease-a4

8 An Interesting Link

"It is not the strongest or the most intelligent who will survive but those who can best manage change."
— Leon C. Megginson, Professor, Louisiana State University

Human Brain: Evolution

According to John Hawks, professor of anthropology at the University of Wisconsin-Madison, "Humans are known for sporting big brains. On average, the size of primates' brains is nearly double what is expected for mammals of comparable body size. Across nearly seven million years, the human brain has tripled in size, with most of this growth occurring in the past two million years."[1] Dr. Hawks explains that our famous ancestor, Lucy (*Australopithecus afarensis*), had a skull with an internal volume of 400–550 mL. This is similar in size to chimpanzee skulls, which hold 400 mL, and slightly less than gorillas, whose skulls have an internal volume of 500–700 mL.

As humans (*Homo sapiens*) evolved, brain size continued to grow. *Homo habilis* is the first member of the *Homo* genus, and lived approximately 1.9 million years ago. *Homo habilis* had a modest increase in brain size, specifically in the regions of the frontal lobe of the brain. This increase in size of the frontal lobes is actually one of the more pronounced differences between humans and mammals of other species. As we discussed at the beginning of this book, the frontal lobes are involved in higher cognitive functions such as thought, planning, problem solving, social engagement, and more. Fossil skulls of *Homo erectus* were found dating back to approximately 1.8 million years ago, and these skulls had brain sizes of approximately 600 mL. As humans evolved, the average brain size increased to over 1,000 mL, and now, *Homo sapiens* have brains of approximately 1,200 mL. This increase in brain size corresponds to the development of increasingly complex societies, language, agricultural technologies, and more.

Throughout evolution, the amount of brain mass related to an animal's or human's total body mass can be expressed by something called an "encephalization quotient" (EQ) and it can actually be calculated with a formula.[2] Among most animal species, a bigger body size results in a bigger brain. However, this relationship is not linear because certain mammals, such as elephants, have a small brain compared to their body mass. The EQ uses cats as the standard, therefore having EQ = 1. The EQ values can be below or above 1, with numbers greater than 1 meaning a relative brain size that is above what is expected. Researchers have found that EQs of 2.5 and 7.5 have been noted in fossils of *Australopithecus afarensis* (3.1–3.6 million years old) and *Homo neanderthalensis* (dating back to 30,000 years ago).[3] Modern humans have the highest EQ of the

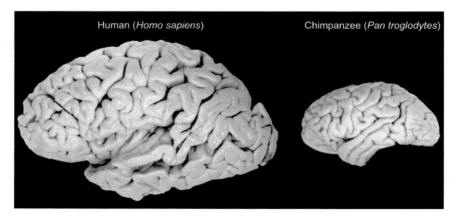

Fig. 8.1. A human brain (left) and a chimpanzee brain (right). Note the similarities but also the stark contrast in size. (Modified from Ref. 5.)

mammals of between 7.4 and 7.8. In other words, the human brain is 7.4- to 7.8-times larger than expected for a mammal weighing as much as we do. Because of the higher EQ number in humans, it is possible that the EQ numbers are linked to intelligence.[4]

But what does the evolution of the human brain have to do with Alzheimer's disease? As humans evolved, the genetic code that was at one point identical across all species concurrently changed. As such, the genetic sequence that codes certain proteins that are uniquely human, as well as proteins that are only found in other species, changed with evolution. For example, both mice and humans produce the amyloid precursor protein (APP) that leads to the β-amyloid-filled plaques in Alzheimer's disease. However, mice have a slightly different version of the APP gene, and thus a slightly different version of the final APP protein. Interestingly, Alzheimer's disease is not seen naturally in aged mice, but it is readily seen in humans. The reason for this could be multifactorial. One possible reason is that the genetic sequence of APP in humans makes the cleaved β-amyloid fragments more susceptible to clumping and forming plaques, while this susceptibility is absent in mice. Another possibility could be that mice simply do not live to be old enough to exhibit Alzheimer's pathology. However, monkeys and apes can live to be 40–60 years old, and although they develop plaques in their brains, they appear to be resistant to Alzheimer's disease. Therefore, it is possible that the specific genetic sequence of β-amyloid in humans may increase our susceptibility to Alzheimer's disease compared to non-human animals.

In order to understand the effects of human β-amyloid in mice, scientists at the University of California, Irvine actually inserted the human β-amyloid gene into mice. This led to the development of plaques within the brain, and the mice exhibited deficits in learning and memory that corresponded to the development of intraneuronal β-amyloid deposits. This transgenic (genetically modified) mouse model of Alzheimer's disease allows scientists to study the development of the pathological features of Alzheimer's disease in an entirely new way.[6]

The reason as to why animals do not develop Alzheimer's disease (unless they are genetically modified to reproduce Alzheimer's pathology) is not entirely clear. It is possible that the specific sequence of the protein in humans makes it more prone to oligomerization. A single β-amyloid protein fragment is known as a monomer, and oligomers are formed when five or more monomers combine. Studies have found that soluble oligomeric β-amyloid is more dangerous than β-amyloid monomers and more harmful than fibrillar β-amyloid (which is a long strand of β-amyloid oligomers).[7-13] Studies in Alzheimer's patients have found that soluble oligomers of β-amyloid are present, in addition to the fibrillar β-amyloid that forms plaques.[14-18] Furthermore, it has been shown that soluble oligomers of β-amyloid that are obtained from the brains of Alzheimer's patients can cause abnormalities in neurons at a 100-fold lower concentration than synthetically formed dimers (two monomers linked together).[19] In fact, it has even been hypothesized that β-amyloid monomers can form "cylinders" called cylindrin molecules, which could even temporarily form pores in the membranes of neurons and destroy the cells.[20,21] Although this cylindrin hypothesis is still being studied, it lends weight to the notion of the damaging properties and neurotoxicity of β-amyloid, suggesting that the effects of β-amyloid can change depending on its structural conformation (i.e. monomer, dimer, oligomer, fibril, or cylindrical).

Three Types of Alzheimer's Disease

Scientists group Alzheimer's disease into three types: early onset, late onset and familial.[22] These groups are not mutually exclusive; familial Alzheimer's disease can (and usually is) early onset. Early-onset Alzheimer's disease has been brought to light in the book-turned-movie *Still Alice*, which is about a renowned linguistics professor who must face early-onset Alzheimer's disease. This form of Alzheimer's is distinguished in terms of the time of diagnosis, namely before the age of 65. The youngest person diagnosed with early-onset Alzheimer's disease was only 17 years old at the time of diagnosis.[23] In fact, there are several families around the world who share an unfortunate mutation that predisposes them to developing Alzheimer's disease in the prime of their lives. Although early-onset Alzheimer's disease is an extremely devastating pathological process, it fortunately accounts for only 5% of individuals living with Alzheimer's disease.[24]

Since early-onset Alzheimer's accounts for such a small population, it is unfortunately often misdiagnosed. Symptoms are often incorrectly attributed to stress or other conflicting diseases. Accurate diagnosis is especially critical so that patients can face their condition and adjust accordingly. This may include scheduling a lighter workload with their employer or rearranging their personal lives with their partners. This seems to be primarily because Alzheimer's disease is commonly known as the old person's disease, so healthcare providers are simply not actively considering it as a differential diagnosis. However, the symptoms of early-onset Alzheimer's are basically identical to the late-onset version. According to data, early-onset Alzheimer's does not progress at a faster rate than its counterpart. There is a perception that it does because the younger age of diagnosis may place the patient in a more difficult position. For instance, early-onset Alzheimer's patients may be admitted at an earlier age into a nursing home, perhaps because their spouses or partners may need to go to work or take care of their children, much more so than older individuals.[24] Moreover, the patient's children, who may still be young, tend to suffer physically and emotionally if their parents can no longer take care of them. Accordingly, there are support groups that are specifically designed for early-onset Alzheimer's. Many Alzheimer's Association support groups offer assistance specifically for children, those with early-onset and early-stage Alzheimer's, and adult caregivers.

Late-onset Alzheimer's is what usually comes to mind when people think of Alzheimer's disease. It is first diagnosed after the age of 65 and may or may not run in families. An interesting hypothesis is the idea that early- and late-onset Alzheimer's disease are different enough to be classified into two distinct subgroups. A 2012 *Frontiers in Neurology* study discussed a dichotomy that was found when administering neuropsychological tests to 280 Alzheimer's patients who were split between the two types. The younger patients exhibited significant impairment in praxis (planning what to do and how to do it) and a tendency for a great impairment in neocortical temporal functions. Patients with late-onset forms had a tendency for worse performances in visual, memory, and orientation, which was associated with abnormalities being more localized to the brain's limbic structures.[25] Although it is extremely unfortunate that familial Alzheimer's disease can affect individuals at such a young age and in such an expected manner, it has helped shed light on the underlying pathological process of the disease and may help us find new ways of treating the disease in the coming years.

Familial Alzheimer's disease is known to be directly linked to genes, with members in at least two generations of a family exhibiting the disease.[26] Familial Alzheimer's disease is also known as early-onset Alzheimer's disease, as it commonly presents itself early in an individual's lifetime. There are three genes that have been linked to familial Alzheimer's disease: *PSEN1*, *PSEN2*, and *APP*.[27] *APP* has been discussed extensively in Chapter 5, but *PSEN1* and *PSEN2* are novel gene discoveries that are linked to the Alzheimer's disease. The gene that is most common in these familial cases of Alzheimer's disease is known as *PSEN1* (on chromosome 14), which codes for a protein known as presenilin-1. This protein normally helps the cell destroy proteins that need to be degraded. However, when the gene is mutated, the cell cannot destroy certain proteins. One of these proteins that cannot be destroyed is known as γ-secretase. This protein is involved in the generation of β-amyloid, and thus when it is overly abundant in the cell, this leads to an increased production of β-amyloid, which increases the formation of the toxic plaques within the brain. Another gene that is implicated in familial Alzheimer's disease is known as *PSEN2* (on chromosome 1), and although it is less prevalent and less studied than *PSEN1*, it has a similar function, and also predisposes individuals with a mutation in *PSEN2* to develop early-onset Alzheimer's disease.

Trisomy 21 (Down Syndrome)

In 1987, researchers were able to find the first gene to be associated with Alzheimer's disease. Out of the 23 pairs of chromosomes in humans, this gene was on chromosome 21. It coded for APP, which is the precursor to β-amyloid. In addition, Down syndrome is also linked to an abnormal feature of chromosome 21: having three copies rather than the standard two copies of the chromosome. Down syndrome is associated with delays in physical and intellectual development. As adults, these individuals typically have mental abilities that are similar to those of an 8-year-old child.[28]

It has also been known that individuals who have Down syndrome are predisposed to develop early-onset Alzheimer's disease in their 30s or 40s (compared to the normal onset of the disease in the sixth and seventh decades of life). To reiterate, Down syndrome is caused by the presence of all or part of a third copy of chromosome 21. This association between having three copies of chromosome 21 in patients with Down syndrome and the early development of Alzheimer's disease lends weight to the idea that making too much APP, and thus too much β-amyloid, can ultimately contribute to the development of Alzheimer's disease. Thus, whenever there are too many copies of the *APP* gene within a cell, there will be an increase in the production of APP. Down syndrome patients are usually diagnosed with Alzheimer's by age 52. On average, death occurs 8 years later. Brain autopsy studies show that by age 40, the brains of almost all individuals who are afflicted with Down syndrome have significant amounts of plaques and tangles, similar to the levels found in Alzheimer's disease patients. Despite these brain changes, not all individuals present symptoms of Alzheimer's disease.[29] It is unclear why researchers have found this disparity. Perhaps it is a diagnosis issue — it is more difficult to differentiate between the cognitive impairments due to Down syndrome and those due to Alzheimer's. However, perhaps there is more to this story.

This serves as an interesting therapeutic target for researchers to focus on — if the production of APP can be dampened, then maybe the production of the toxic proteins that accumulate in Alzheimer's can be mitigated. On the other hand, however, the normal production of APP is actually beneficial to normal cell functioning. It is the abnormal, uncontrolled, and unregulated overproduction of APP and the ensuing β-amyloid that can be damaging.

Since the discovery of the *APP* gene on chromosome 21, Alzheimer's disease has been better characterized as a polygenic disease. In other words, the development of the disease is due to a multitude of genes that interact with one another in varying and unpredictable ways. Unlike certain disorders that are linked to a single gene, such as Huntington's disease, Alzheimer's disease is linked to many genes, each of which may contribute only a small amount to the development of the disease, but exhibiting additive and synergistic interactions with one another.

The Interesting Role of Sleep in Alzheimer's Disease

Sleep is an incredibly important aspect of normal health, and has even been implicated in Alzheimer's disease. Recent studies have shown that sleep duration and sleep position both play critical roles in the elimination of toxins, such as β-amyloid, from the brain.[30-32] These studies support the idea that sleep serves a critical function, which is not surprising, since sleep is a conserved trait of all animal species. In 2009, a collaboration between Washington University and Stanford University sought out bodily functions and processes that are responsible for regulating the production and clearance of the Alzheimer's disease hallmark, β-amyloid protein. In their quest, they identified lack of sleep as a crucial component in the advancement of Alzheimer's disease. By inserting probes into the brains of mice with Alzheimer's disease, researchers were able to calculate the amount of β-amyloid protein within the fluid-filled space surrounding the neurons (known as the interstitial space). Their calculations indicated a strong correlation between wakefulness and β-amyloid protein concentration.

Not only did they notice a decreased β-amyloid protein concentration in the interstitial space after a night of restful sleep, but they also observed significant increases in β-amyloid protein concentration even with short periods of sleep deprivation. These results suggested chronic sleep deprivation as a culprit of β-amyloid plaque build-up, therefore suggesting this as a possible cause of Alzheimer's disease; however, they had not specifically identified a mechanism by which the brain clears β-amyloid during sleep.

It was not until 2013 that a study conducted at the University of Rochester and New York University further investigated the role of sleep in Alzheimer's disease. This new research identified the glymphatic system, a sleep-dependent waste-clearing pathway of the brain, as the exact process by which β-amyloid protein and other toxins are flushed out of the brain. The authors indicated that when individuals are asleep or, interestingly, anesthetized, the brain stays fully active in order to clean out the toxins that have accumulated during daily processes. In order to clean the brain, the supportive glial brain cells that surround neurons shrink and therefore increase the size (volume) of the interstitial space by 60%. This increase in the interstitial space allows for an inflow of cerebrospinal fluid (clear liquid surrounding the brain) from channels beside the arteries, which exchanges with the already-present fluid and, by doing so, physically clears the β-amyloid and other toxins that are present inside the interstitial space. Conversely, when an individual is awake, the interstitial space is much smaller than while asleep; therefore, CSF cannot flow freely and reach deep within the brain, and thus clearance of β-amyloid and other toxins occurs at half the rate. These results suggest that sleep is an extremely important function that helps remove toxic components from the brain, indicating that sleep quality plays an essential role in the development and progression of Alzheimer's disease.

A more recent study published in the *Journal of Neurobiology of Disease* in 2015 further explored the intricacy and association of sleep and Alzheimer's disease.[32] Researchers from Stony Brooks University anesthetized mice and used functional magnetic resonance imaging (FMRI) alongside other highly advanced imaging techniques in order to understand and validate the efficiency of the glymphatic system (mentioned above) in various sleeping positions. They injected mice with neurotoxins and placed them on their sides, stomachs, and backs and compared the rates at which CSF could fill the interstitial space and clear out toxins during anesthetized sleep. Their results indicated that sleeping on one's side (see Fig. 8.2), as opposed to other positions, more effectively removes brain waste, specifically β-amyloid. So far, the researchers have not been able to fully explain why the glymphatic system works more efficiently while sleeping on one's side, for it may depend on multiple physiological processes. For example, different head, and body positions cause stretching in the head and neck vasculature, and nerves, which has varying effects on blood flow and CSF flow.

In conclusion, sleep is unequivocally one of the most essential restorative measures of any animal, including human beings. Just as a city requires a sewage and waste management system, our brains require sleep in order to stay clean and function properly. This is specifically true for those who are at risk of or are suffering from neurodegenerative disorders such as Alzheimer's disease. However, in order for one to fully reap the benefits of this cleansing process, it must be unaided (without the use of drugs such as melatonin), uninterrupted, regular, and preferably in the lateral position (on one's side).

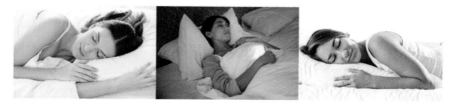

Fig. 8.2. A study by Stony Brook University suggests that the lateral position of sleeping on one's side (compared to other positions such as sleeping on one's back or stomach) proved most effective for clearing toxins from the brain via the glymphatic system. (Figure credit: Ref. 33.)

References

1. http://www.scientificamerican.com/article/how-has-human-brain-evolved/

2. Jerison HJ. (1973) *Evolution of the Brain and Intelligence*. New York, NY: Academic Press.

3. Marino L. (1998) A comparison of encephalization between odontocete cetaceans and anthropoid primates. *Brain Behav Evol* **51**: 230–238.

4. DeFelipe J. (2011) The evolution of the brain, the human nature of cortical circuits, and intellectual creativity. *Front Neuroanat* **5**: 29.

5. https://commons.wikimedia.org/wiki/Gyri#/media/File:Human_and_chimp_brain.png

6. Oddo S, Caccamo A, Shepherd JD, *et al*. (2003) Triple-transgenic model of Alzheimer's disease with plaques and tangles: Intracellular Aβ and synaptic dysfunction. *Neuron* **39**(3): 409–421.

7. http://www.ncbi.nlm.nih.gov/pmc/articles/PMC3563737/

8. Selkoe DJ. (2008) Soluble oligomers of the amyloid beta-protein impair synaptic plasticity and behavior. *Behav Brain Res* **192**(1): 106–113.

9. Wang HW, Pasternak JF, Kuo H, *et al*. (2002) Soluble oligomers of beta amyloid (1–42) inhibit long-term potentiation but not long-term depression in rat dentate gyrus. *Brain Res* **924**(2): 133–140.

10. Lambert MP, Barlow AK, Chromy BA, *et al*. (1998) Diffusible, nonfibrillarligands derived from Abeta1–42 are potent central nervous system neurotoxins. *Proc Natl Acad Sci USA* **95**(11): 6448–6453.

11. Kayed R, Head E, Thompson JL, *et al*. (2003) Common structure of soluble amyloid oligomers implies common mechanism of pathogenesis. *Science* **300**(5618): 486–489.

12. Dahlgren KN, Manelli AM, Stine WB Jr, *et al*. (2002) Oligomeric and fibrillar species of amyloid-beta peptides differentially affect neuronal viability. *J Biol Chem* **277**(35): 32046–32053.

13. Ono K, Condron MM, Teplow DB. (2009) Structure-neurotoxicity relationships of amyloid beta-protein oligomers. *Proc Natl Acad Sci USA* **106**(35): 14745–14750.

14. Townsend M, Shankar GM, Mehta T, *et al*. (2006) Effects of secreted oligomers of amyloid beta-protein on hippocampal synaptic plasticity: A potent role for trimers. *J Physiol* **572**(Pt 2): 477–492.

15. Walsh DM, Klyubin I, Fadeeva JV, *et al.* (2002) Naturally secreted oligomers of amyloid beta protein potently inhibit hippocampal long-term potentiation *in vivo. Nature* **416**(6880): 535–539.

16. Shankar GM, Li S, Mehta TH, *et al.* (2008) Amyloid-beta protein dimers isolated directly from Alzheimer's brains impair synaptic plasticity and memory. *Nat Med* **14**(8): 837–842.

17. Cleary JP, Walsh DM, Hofmeister JJ, *et al.* (2005) Natural oligomers of the amyloid-beta protein specifically disrupt cognitive function. *Nat Neurosci* **8**(1): 79–84.

18. Lesne S, Koh MT, Kotilinek L, *et al.* (2006) A specific amyloid-beta protein assembly in the brain impairs memory. *Nature* **440**(7082): 352–357.

19. Jin M, Shepardson N, Yang T, *et al.* (2011) Soluble amyloid beta-protein dimers isolated from Alzheimer cortex directly induce tau hyperphosphorylation and neuritic degeneration. *Proc Natl Acad Sci USA* **108**(14): 5819–5824.

20. https://www.researchgate.net/publication/277078789_Comparative_modeling_of_hypothetical_amyloid_pores_based_on_cylindrin

21. http://science.sciencemag.org/content/335/6073/1228

22. http://www.livestrong.com/article/27347-early-onset-symptoms-alzheimers/

23. http://www.nia.nih.gov/alzheimers/publication/preventing-alzheimers-disease/risk-factors-alzheimers-disease

24. Mayo Clinic staff. *Early-Onset Alzheimer's: When Symptoms Begin Before 65.* Mayo Clinic.

25. Sá F, Pinto P, Cunha C, *et al.* (2012) Differences between early and late-onset Alzheimer's disease in neuropsychological tests. *Front Neurol* **3**: 81.

26. http://www.webmd.com/alzheimers/guide/alzheimers-types

27. Younkin SG. (1998) The *APP* and *PS1/2* mutations linked to early onset familial Alzheimer's disease increase the extracellular concentration of Aβ1–42 (43). *Presenilins Alzheimers Dis* 27–33.

28. Malt EA, Dahl RC, Haugsand TM, *et al.* (2013) Health and disease in adults with Down syndrome. *Tidsskr Nor Laegeforen* **133**(3): 290–294.

29. http://www.emedicinehealth.com/alzheimers_disease_in__down_syndrome/page3_em.htm

30. Kang J-E, Lim MM, Bateman RJ, *et al.* (2009) Amyloid-β dynamics are regulated by orexin and the sleep–wake cycle. *Science* **326**(5955): 1005–1007.

31. Mendelsohn AR, Larrick JW. (2013) Sleep facilitates clearance of metabolites from the brain: Glymphatic function in aging and neurodegenerative diseases. *Rejuvenation Res* **16**(6): 518–523.

32. Lee H, Xie L, Yu M, *et al.* (2015) The effect of body posture on brain glymphatic transport. *J Neurosci* **35**(31): 11034–11044.

33. http://sb.cc.stonybrook.edu/news/general/150804sleeping.php

Part II
Novel Therapies
and Future Directions

9
Surgical Treatments for Dementia

"Only the ideas that we actually live are of any value."
— *Demian: The Story of Emil Sinclair's Youth* by Hermann Hesse,
Nobel Laureate (Literature, 1946)

This chapter of the book on surgical treatments will begin not with a particular surgical solution, but rather a question. The question arose from a surgical proposal from the 1970s for an 84-year-old dementia-stricken man. This man's incessant yelling caused him to be unmanageable in all settings, whether it was in his private home with his aged wife or in a hospital facility. The proposal suggested removing one of the nerves supplying the patient's vocal cords, changing his voice to "a very acceptable soft tone." At the time, the proposal was suggested and unanimously endorsed by an *ad hoc* advisory committee consisting of psychiatrists, internal medicine physicians, Ear, Nose and Throat (ENT) surgeons, and other staff members at the hospital where the patient was admitted. Although conflicted, the patient's wife maintained that her husband himself would have wanted the surgery. Ultimately, the hospital's Department of Surgery did not allow the surgery on the terms that it involved some risk and was a non-medical operation. Dr. George Robertson, from the Department of Anaesthetics at the Royal Infirmary in Scotland, brings a different perspective on why this surgical proposal was to be rejected. He asked whether a treatment such as the one proposed above would effectively help improve the patient's general condition. He related this treatment to the treatment of the recurrent pneumonias that an Alzheimer's patient is very likely to contract.[1] How many recurrent pneumonia infections do you treat when an Alzheimer's patient is likely to contract it again? Should there be a limit?

The complexity of the 1970 surgical treatment to address only one aspect of dementia foreshadows the multifaceted difficulty of this problem. Alzheimer's disease causes a variety of medical problems, and as important as it is to treat the effects of Alzheimer's disease, it may be more effective to find a cure for the source of these issues in the first place. We need a treatment for the illness, not just its symptoms. We will now explore clinical trials — old and new — that set out to solve precisely this problem.

Introduction to Neurosurgery and the "Miraculous" Cures of Dementia in Select Disorders

Although there are many different academic fields that focus on studying the brain and that approach it from different perspectives, they are unanimously attempting to uncover the mysteries that the brain holds. Various fields such as neurobiology, psychology, cognitive science, and neurology all focus on understanding the brain, but from different perspectives. The field of neurosurgery seeks to understand the brain in the most direct way possible, to actually expose it, manipulate it, and see what happens. Some of the earlier neurosurgical experiments that attempted to directly uncover the mysteries of the brain involved taking an electrode and actually touching different parts of the brain to see what happens. This resulted in landmark discoveries. One of the parts of the cortex (the surface of the brain) that was discovered via this method is known as the motor cortex. The motor cortex is responsible for moving different parts of the body. Interestingly, the right motor cortex is responsible for moving the left side of the body, and vice versa, so when neurosurgeons stimulated the motor cortex on the right side of the brain, they could elicit a response on the opposite, or contralateral, side of the body. For example, by touching a specific part of the motor cortex, the patient's arm, leg, mouth, or body would move. This was the basis for how intraoperative neurosurgical experimentation could uncover what parts of the brain were responsible for what. The classical case studies of various patients who had damage to various parts of their cortex allowed scientists and physicians to understand the general roles that the frontal lobe or the hippocampus played, as in the cases of Phineas Gage or Patient H.M.

Phineas Gage was a railroad worker who, in an unfortunate accident, had a massive spike blow through his skull. This destroyed the front part of his brain. Miraculously, he survived, and was able to recover from this accident. His close friends and family soon discovered, however, that Mr. Gage no longer had the same upbeat personality that he used to have. They began to realize that he had fundamentally changed — he had become "different." This led scientists to realize that the frontal lobe (the very front part of your brain) is involved in personality and complex cognitive tasks. Damage or destruction to this part of the brain leads to personality changes, difficulty with executive functioning, and difficulty planning. It also leads to a changes in temperament and a lack of inhibition.

Another interesting patient that greatly contributed to the field of neuroscience is a patient known as H.M. Patient H.M. suffered from intractable seizures. In order to treat these seizures, neurosurgeons decided to remove the part of the brain from which the seizures were originating, known as the foci of the seizures. Unfortunately, the foci originated in an area of the brain known as the hippocampus. The hippocampus is crucial for memory formation, and when both hippocampi were removed from H.M., he lost the ability to form new memories. This was an incredible case that allowed scientists and physicians to decipher the role of the hippocampus in memory.

These cases are just a few of the many fascinating examples of how we began to understand how the brain works. Our collective understanding of the brain is still in its infancy, and there is so much more to learn. With new imaging techniques, electrophysiological recording, and clinical intuition, we are beginning to unearth the secrets of the brain, but there is so much more to learn.

Surgical Clinical Trials: The Ventriculo-Peritoneal (UP) Shunt Trial

There is a high demand to explore these different avenues for Alzheimer's disease; in fact, if no new medicines are found to prevent or delay the progression of Alzheimer's disease, the number of afflicted in the United States will reach 13.5 million by the year 2050 (Alzheimer's Association). With the development of novel medical technologies, there is potential of surgical treatments for Alzheimer's disease that may include the use of shunts, devices, and stem cell injections in order to palliate the disease.

Cerebrospinal fluid (CSF) shunts have been used for decades to treat hydrocephalus as a way of clearing toxic species from the body.[2] The premise of a shunt treatment is to remove the toxic factors that may accumulate in the CSF of an Alzheimer's disease patient. The toxic factors may include β-amyloid protein fragments and abnormally altered tau proteins, the two archetypical toxins of an Alzheimer's-afflicted brain. A shunt treatment is hypothesized to reverse the detrimental changes to the brain by draining out those toxic elements and allowing the CSF to be replenished. One device under clinical trial is COGNIShunt, a ventriculo-peritoneal shunt that drains CSF from the skull and into the abdominal cavity. This device differs from shunts for treating hydrocephalus only in that it has been engineered to allow for lower drainage of the CSF.[3] Research results on the COGNIShunt from a Phase I/II pilot clinical trial by Baxter Healthcare were published in *Neurology* in October 2002.[4] Patients with mild-to-moderate Alzheimer's disease participated in the study: 15 were randomly selected to receive the shunt implantation and 14 people received no investigational treatment. The primary objective of this pilot study was to assess the safety of the shunt procedure. This preliminary study, despite having a very small sample size, showed encouraging data regarding stabilization of mental function in the shunted patients, as scored on the Mattis Dementia Rating Scale. In October 2003, the developer of COGNIShunt, Eunoe, Inc. (a San Francisco-based medical device company), began conducting more clinical trials at the Cleveland Clinic Foundation in order to assess the safety and effectiveness of the treatment and to test the hypothesis that the toxic factors in CSF contribute to the destruction of brain cells in Alzheimer's disease. On June 14, 2004, the study was closed based on the results of both a first and second interim analysis, which showed there was not sufficient evidence to demonstrate efficacy in support of US pre-market approval of the device.[5]

Stem Cell Trials: Pre-clinical Data and Clinical Trials

Stem cells are special cells that have the potential to become any cell in the body. Their power lies in the ability to transform a naïve stem cell into a specific cell type that is normal and healthy and is able to do whatever you want it to do. For example, in Type I diabetes, there is a defective population of cells within the pancreas, known as β-islet cells. These cells normally function by secreting a hormone known as insulin. Insulin is basically a molecule that allows cells to take sugar that is floating in the blood and bring it inside the cell so that the sugar can be broken down and used for energy. When patients develop Type I diabetes, they do not have any β-islet cells in their pancreas, and therefore cannot take up sugar from their blood in order to use it for energy production. This quickly becomes a significant and even deadly problem if appropriate medications, mainly the introduction of insulin, are not initiated. One of the potential uses of stem cell therapies is to actually grow, using the patient's own stem cells, β-islet cells that can then be transplanted into that patient's pancreas. This is the idea behind stem cell therapies: to grow the cell type of interest that may be missing or damaged within the patient's body, and reintroduce a population of normal cells in order to fix a disease state.

One extremely interesting development in the field of stem cell therapeutics has been the idea of induced pluripotent stem cells (iPSCs).

Classically, stem cells that are pluripotent, meaning that they can become any cell within the body, were derived from human embryos. This is fraught with ethical controversy, as the formation of normal pluripotent stem cells necessitated the destruction of a human embryo. In 2006, Dr. Shinya Yamanaka showed that normal, fully differentiated human cells can be reprogrammed into pluripotent cells via the introduction of a certain set of molecular factors.[6] He was eventually awarded the Nobel Prize in 2012 for this work. The use of iPSCs effectively circumvents the ethical problems associated with the classical creation of pluripotent stem cells, while maintaining the therapeutic power that pluripotent stem cells hold. Now, iPSC technology can be used to take skin cells from a patient with Type I diabetes, and those skin cells can be reprogrammed back into pluripotent stem cells. Those pluripotent stem cells can then be converted into β-islet cells and then transplanted back into that patient's pancreas in order to theoretically cure Type I diabetes. This is the general idea in theory, but practically, there are many problems that must be dealt with, such as how to ensure that the transplanted cells survive, how to ensure that the cells do not form a tumor, and so on. These specific problems are currently being worked on by researchers and physicians around the world. Many other diseases could potentially be impacted by stem cell therapies, including Parkinson's disease, blunt spinal cord trauma, stroke, retinal damage, cancer, and many more. As we discover more about stem cell science and biology, learn more about how to effectively grow and culture cells, and develop newer and better alternatives to transplant the cells and allow them to survive within the body for a prolonged period of time, the potential for using stem cells in order to treat and cure diseases is increasingly becoming a reality. Fortunately, one of the most promising prospects for the treatment of Alzheimer's disease lies within stem cell-based therapies.

There are currently no Food and Drug Administration (FDA)-approved stem cell therapies for Alzheimer's. However, there is huge potential for avant-garde stem cell therapies to benefit the Alzheimer's brain in various ways, such as helping modulate inflammation, stimulating re-myelination, and supplying trophic support. "This may enhance the life of dying neurons," suggests Mahendra Rao, leader of the New York Stem Cell Foundation Research Institute.[7] One example is the initial work of StemGenex, a company that is studying the effects of adipose-derived stem cells and their ability to assist in rebuilding lost nerve fibers, rather than replacing them with healthy neurons. StemGenex is currently studying the effectiveness of mesenchymal stem cell therapy in patients with both early- and late-stage Alzheimer's disease.[8]

In addition to stem cell-based surgical therapies, one novel approach to the treatment of Alzheimer's disease is the transposition of the omentum onto the brains of patients with Alzheimer's disease. Omental transposition surgery was conducted on six patients with biopsy-confirmed Alzheimer's disease. The omentum is an organ that is located within the abdominal (peritoneal) cavity that covers, protects, and nourishes the abdominal organs. It has an extremely rich blood (vascular) and lymphatic vessel supply. This means that the omentum can nourish an organ, as well as remove toxic waste and metabolic products from that organ. When parts of the omentum were transposed (moved) onto the brains of patients with Alzheimer's disease, researchers found improvements in the cognition, function, and behavior of patients for up to 3.5 years after transplantation.[9]

According to Dr. Harry Goldsmith, a pioneer in omental transposition surgery, the physiological characteristics of the omentum include absorption of excess fluid (edema), inhibition of fibrosis and scarring, penetration of the blood–brain barrier, and formation of new blood vessels.[10] Omental transposition surgery appears to be a potentially useful tool in the treatment of Alzheimer's disease. Although the exact molecular mechanisms underlying the benefits of omental transplants onto the brains of individuals with Alzheimer's disease are unknown, they are thought to be mediated in part by the formation of new blood vessels and the clearance of excess fluid and waste products from the brain via lymphatic drainage.

Omental transposition surgery offers a lot of hope for the future, and has become increasingly accepted as a clinical tool for patients, even those who are suffering from spinal cord injuries. Spinal cord injuries have been effectively treated in China and in other countries around the world, with some function being restored in patients.[11] The transposition of omental tissue onto the brains of patients with Alzheimer's disease is primarily performed by neurosurgeons, but requires the movement of omental tissue towards the brain by general surgeons. The procedure involves the creation of an incision in the abdominal wall in order to retrieve the omentum, which is highly vascularized fatty tissue that is approximately 14 inches long. The omentum resembles an apron that drapes over the intestines and other organs within the abdominal cavity. Once removed, the omentum is then lengthened and tunneled underneath the skin, and run through the chest and neck, eventually reaching the head. Once the omentum is near the brain, the neurosurgeon performs a craniotomy (creation of a bone flap) and secure the omentum onto the brain. The omentum sits underneath the dura mater, directly on the side of the brain itself, and is secured in place by suturing the dura over the omentum.[12]

Currently, a clinical trial led by Dr. Danniel Cottam is underway at the Bariatric Medicine Institute in Salt Lake City, Utah. The trial will enroll up to 25 patients and is investigating the safety and effectiveness of omental transposition in patients with early-stage Alzheimer's disease. These new surgical approaches represent an exciting time for Alzheimer's disease therapy explorations; we are actively pursuing treatments for Alzheimer's, as well as symptomatic treatments. The question posed in the beginning of this chapter — how much is too much? — is less of a problem. As we test the efficacy and safety of surgical treatments for Alzheimer's disease, we can only hope that the source of Alzheimer's disease is being attacked, rather than just its symptoms.

Deep-Brain Stimulation

Another approach to the treatment of Alzheimer's disease is electrical stimulation. One example in which an electrode can actually treat a disease is the neurodegenerative disorder known as PD. PD is another well-known disorder in which a certain subset of cells within the brain dies out. These cells are responsible for producing and secreting dopamine, which is an important neurotransmitter within the brain, and they are involved in the various circuits within the brain that control movement. As these cells die, the patient begins to develop movement disorders, mainly tremors. The movement disorders progress as the disease process ensues, and eventually, there is a complete lack of dopamine. This usually leads to death if not controlled by medications or other therapies. Fortunately, Parkinson's disease is very amenable to pharmacological treatments. There are several drugs that work in an excellent fashion in order to control and manage the disease for many years after diagnosis. Additionally, there is a surgical procedure known as deep-brain stimulation (DBS) that can be used to treat later-stage PD, which works extremely well. In this procedure, surgeons place a small electrode deep within the brain. The electrode is able to stimulate specific brain regions and actually terminate the debilitating tremors associated with PD. This approach has been tested in Alzheimer's disease, and may eventually play a role in the treatment regimen of advanced Alzheimer's disease. In the case of Alzheimer's disease, specific neural networks and brain regions that are intimately involved in memory formation and consolidation, such as the hippocampus, may one day be targeted by electrical stimulation in order to enhance those specific circuits. A clinical trial is underway,[13] focusing on evaluating the safety of the DBS of a structure within the brain known as the fornix in individuals with mild Alzheimer's disease. Results from a separate study evaluating DBS in memory circuits in order to treat Alzheimer's found that impaired glucose utilization within the brain could be reversed, with suggestions of improvements in cognitive performance in some patients.[14] This study was a Phase I clinical trial, however, and such trials are primarily designed to evaluate the safety of the procedure.[15]

In general, the most promising approaches for the treatment of Alzheimer's disease appear to deal with supplementing the brain's natural ability to heal and protect itself, while negating any adverse side effects that the drug or therapy may be associated with.

References

1. Gafner G. (1987) Surgery to quieten the yelling of a demented old man. *J Med Ethics* **13**(4): 195–197.

2. May C, Kaye JA, Atack JR, *et al.* (1990) Cerebrospinal fluid production is reduced in healthy aging. *Neurology* **40**(3 Pt 1): 500–503.

3. Silverberg GD, Mayo M, Saul T, *et al.* (2004) Novel ventriculo-peritoneal shunt in Alzheimer's disease cerebrospinal fluid biomarkers. *Expert Rev Neurother* **4**: 97–107.

4. Silverberg GD, Levinthal E, Sullivan EV, *et al.* (2002) Assessment of low-flow CSF drainage as a treatment for AD: Results of a randomized pilot study. *Neurology* **59**: 1139–1145.

5. http://globenewswire.com/news-release/2005/09/29/334180/87040/en/Integra-LifeSciences-Acquires-Eunoe-Inc-s-Intellectual-Property-Estate.html

6. http://en.wikipedia.org/wiki/Induced-pluripotent-stem-cell

7. http://www.alzforum.org/news/conference-coverage/ready-or-not-stem-cell therapies-poised-enter-trials-alzheimers

8. https://stemgenex.com/studies/alzheimers-stem-cell-studies

9. Shankle WR, Hara J, Blomsen L, *et al.* (2008) Omentum transposition surgery for patients with Alzheimer's disease: A case series. *Neurol Res* **30**(3): 313–325.

10. Goldsmith HS. (2004) The evolution of omentum transposition: From lymphedema to spinal cord, stroke and Alzheimer's disease. *Neurol Res* **26**(5): 586–593.

11. http://www.sci-therapies.info/omentum.htm

12. https://clinicaltrials.gov/ct2/show/NCT02349191

13. https://www.nia.nih.gov/alzheimers/clinical-trials/advance-deep-brain-stimulation-patients-mild-probable-alzheimers-disease

14. https://sites.oxy.edu/clint/physio/article/APhaseITrialofDeepBrainStimula-tionofmemorycircuitsinalheimers.pdf

15. http://www.ncbi.nlm.nih.gov/pubmed/?term=dbs-f+alzheimers

10 Is There a Link to Traumatic Brain Injury?

"Discovery consists of looking at the same thing as everyone else and thinking something different."

— Albert Szent-Györgyi, Nobel Laureate (Physiology or Medicine, 1937)

A common question that arises is whether or not traumatic brain injury (TBI) or concussion can lead to Alzheimer's disease. Indeed, there has been much recent coverage in the press regarding the effect of repetitive concussions on the brain. First, to clarify, a TBI includes any type of injury to the head. This may be severe with hemorrhages (bleeds) and coma, or it may be mild. Mild TBIs are very common and include concussions, which are defined as any transient change in sensorium after an impact to the body. Sensorium refers to the perception of the body's senses, and includes the sensation of consciousness. The impact does not necessarily have to hit the head, and there does not have to be a loss of consciousness.[1,2] Patients sometimes describe a mild TBI, or concussion, as "stars before their eyes" or a being in a "daze" after the injury. Conservative estimates place the number of emergency room visits for TBI to be in excess of 2.1 million per year in the United States. The majority of these are for mild TBI or concussions.[3] There has been a great deal of interest in concussion in young athletes. The fastest-growing category of TBI in the civilian population, however, is occurring in the population over the age of 65. These patients may suffer a mild TBI from a ground-level fall. This presents a particular problem to the medical field, as these folks often have comorbidities and a diminished reserve for tolerating a TBI.[4,5]

The symptoms of concussion include, but are not limited to, headaches, nausea/vomiting, disequilibrium, blurred vision, memory lapses, and trouble with thinking or focusing. Clearly, this suggests that there is altered brain function.[6,7] Alarmingly, the brain chemistry and metabolism is altered after a concussion, putting the brain in a vulnerable state. Another impact, even if it is very mild, can lead to the serious and fatal (in 50% of cases) second impact syndrome. This is characterized by rapid cerebral edema (brain swelling) and herniation (where the brain actually pushes out through the skull) often within minutes of the second impact.[8,9] The reported cases of this have usually been in younger patients and related to sports injuries. Recent guidelines have been established regarding the diagnosis of concussion, and new laws have been enacted as to when an athlete may return to play after a concussion. How long do the post-concussive symptoms (post-concussive syndrome) last? A concussion may be transient, but may also last for 6–8 weeks. It is not uncommon in our TBI and concussion clinic at the Neurotrauma Center at the University of California, Irvine to have patients with complaints 2–3 months after their injury. The symptoms may be subtle. For example, patients may describe their thinking as being slowed, although on our routine physical examination, no abnormalities may be detected.

The conventional imaging studies of computed tomography or magnetic resonance imaging (MRI) scans of patients with concussion are usually normal and do not show any acute processes. This is likely because these imaging modalities are not sensitive enough to detect the swelling that is occurring in the brain. Newer studies with MRI scans suggest that specific imaging of the fiber tracts may show focal swelling and injury that is consistent with the post-concussive symptoms.[10,11] Currently, it is difficult and expensive to perform these newer MRI scans on an acute clinical basis, and most of these studies are done on a research basis. In the future, it is likely that newer techniques will be developed. Interestingly, there has been a great deal of interest in identifying specific biomarkers that may be obtained from the blood in order to detect TBI. Biomarkers for concussion are specific substances, usually proteins, that are elevated after the injury. Ideally, these would correlate with the degree of the injury and would have some predictive value that could guide therapy.[12–14]

Concussion is the mildest form of TBI; nonetheless, it clearly has effects on brain function, as manifested by the symptoms we discussed above. A question that arises is whether concussion has a long-term impact on the brain. We have discussed the rare case of the second impact syndrome, but what about the patient that rides out the course of the concussion and returns to normal? It has been well established that immediately after the primary concussive force (the primary injury), there is a complex cascade of cellular events that occurs in the brain. Among these is the release of excitotoxins, which are substances from the neurons themselves that affect the influx of calcium and water into the cell, thus contributing to swelling. There is also the activation of an inflammatory response resulting from the migration of microglia cells into the area of injury.[15,16] These microglia cells reside in the brain and are the equivalent of the macrophages or white blood cells in the blood. They are responsible for immune defense.

The injured brain is exquisitely sensitive to secondary injuries. These may occur if the brain has inadequate blood flow (ischemia) or oxygen (hypoxia), and may come about from external forces on the body. This is why in our neurotrauma centers there is such great effort spent on maintaining the homeostasis of the patient. Additionally, the ischemia and hypoxia may occur as a result of the local swelling and inflammatory processes. Furthermore, hypoxia and ischemia have been shown to increase the deposition of the amyloid proteins.[17]

It should come as no surprise that a single episode of head injury may have distant sequelae such as the loss of the normal grey and white matter densities years after the injury. Grey matter refers to the part of the brain that is composed of cell bodies, while white matter is the part of the brain that contains myelinated axons. Pathological studies of patients that sustained a single documented TBI and survived (10 hours to 47 years) demonstrated an increased amount of β-amyloid plaques and neurofibrillary tangles when compared to age-matched controls. There was a correlation between the severity of the TBI and the prevalence of the plaques. The finding of β-amyloid plaques appearing within hours of a TBI has led to the hypothesis that the injury initiates β-amyloid plaque formation, which then catalyzes the further accumulation of the amyloid precursor protein in the damaged neurons. The balance between the formation of β-amyloid and its breakdown is disturbed and biased towards the accumulation of the protein.[18-21] Although there are epidemiological studies that show an association between Alzheimer's disease and TBI, not all of the patients who have β-amyloid plaques pathologically demonstrate the signs and symptoms of Alzheimer's. Clearly, there are other genetic and biological factors that come into play, and further research is being conducted on the molecular pathways and processes that lead from TBI to Alzheimer's disease.

Chronic Traumatic Encephalopathy

We have seen how a single episode of TBI can lead to one of the hallmarks of Alzheimer's disease: the amyloid plaque. What is the effect of multiple concussions? The effect of literally hundreds to thousands of concussions on the brain has been studied in boxers. The term "dementia pugilistica" has been applied to the dementia and constellation of symptoms that career boxers are prone to demonstrating. The symptoms are insidious and include irritability, aggressive attitude, poor impulse control, short-term memory loss, depression, and suicidal ideation.[22-24] These symptoms may occur after a latent phase that may last from several years to several decades. Recently, this has been recognized to occur in other contact sports wherein frequent mild TBIs or concussions occur. Included in these sports is American football and ice hockey. Many of the neuropathological studies in this area have been conducted on retired National Football League (NFL) players.

A more modern nomenclature for this is chronic traumatic encephalopathy (CTE).[25,26]

The neuropathological findings of CTE have been well characterized. One of the principle findings is the accumulation of phosphorylated tau proteins in neurons and astrocytes. Tau's pattern and distribution in the brain are unique in CTE and different from other tauopathies, including Alzheimer's disease. The tau proteins are found in the neurofibrillary tangles. Early in the disease, these tangles found in the regions around the blood vessels. As the disease progresses further, there is involvement of the superficial layers of the nearby cortex. Not all cases of CTE have amyloid plaques. In autopsy studies, 30–40% of the CTE patients had both amyloid plaques and neurofibrillary tangles. In the late phase, there is widespread involvement of the temporal lobe, thalamus, and brainstem.[27,28] The molecular mechanisms underlying the development of neurofibrillary tangles and the deposition of phosphorylated tau proteins are areas of intense research. In a mouse model of repetitive concussion, Petraglia and colleagues have demonstrated that there is a tremendous inflammatory response with the influx of microglia after a TBI. With a single concussion, there was an acute, reactive astrocytosis that did not persist past 6 months. Some have postulated that frequent concussions lead to the influx of calcium, which, via a cascade of enzymes, leads to the hyper-phosphorylation of tau proteins. These proteins are normally involved in the normal architecture of the cell. With hyper-phosphorylation, the tau proteins misfold and form aggregates, which then contribute to the formation of neurofibrillary tangles.[29–32]

TBI in the Military

It has recently been recognized that as many as 300,000 recent US veterans of the Iraq and Afghanistan conflicts may have suffered a TBI. These range from concussions to blast injuries from the improvised explosive devices. Neuropathological studies on a few of these veterans who have expired have demonstrated findings that are very similar to

CTE. It seems that a blast injury may start a cascade of events that leads to the abnormal accumulation of tau proteins.[33,34] A better understanding of the injury mechanism may provide us with improved approaches to treating the frequent clinical complaints that accompany blast injuries: post-concussive syndrome, post-traumatic stress disorder, post-traumatic headache, and CTE.[35,36] Further studies need to be conducted on the long-term effects of these injuries on veterans.

Epidemiological studies have demonstrated that there is a relationship between TBI and Alzheimer's disease. It is clear that the cascade of neuronal injury and inflammation may be started with a mild TBI or concussion. This can lead to the development of one of the key hallmarks of Alzheimer's disease: β-amyloid plaques. How this proliferates and spreads and whether this ultimately results in clinical Alzheimer's disease are areas of intense research. CTE is clearly associated with a history of multiple concussions. This leads to a dementia that is similar to but different from that of Alzheimer's. The predominant pathology with CTE is the finding of tau proteins in neurofibrillary tangles. Understanding the mechanisms regarding how these accumulate and lead to the symptomatology of CTE is an area of continued study.

References

1. Provance AJ, Engelman GH, Terhune EB, Coel RA. (2016) Management of sport-related concussion in the pediatric and adolescent population. *Orthopedics* **39**: 24–30.
2. Shetty T, Raince A, Manning E, Tsiouris AJ. (2016) Imaging in chronic traumatic encephalopathy and traumatic brain injury. *Sports Health* **8**: 26–36.
3. Coronado VG, McGuire LC, Sarmiento K, *et al.* (2012) Trends in traumatic brain injury in the U.S. and the public health response: 1995–2009. *J Safety Res* **43**: 299–307.
4. Cuthbert JP, Corrigan JD, Whiteneck GG, *et al.* (2012) Extension of the representativeness of the Traumatic Brain Injury Model Systems National Database: 2001 to 2010. *J Head Trauma Rehabil* **27**: E15–E27.

5. Pearson WS, Sugerman DE, McGuire LC, Coronado VG. (2012) Emergency department visits for traumatic brain injury in older adults in the United States: 2006–2008. *West J Emerg Med* **13**: 289–293.

6. Marshall S, Bayley M, McCullagh S, *et al.* (2015) Updated clinical practice guidelines for concussion/mild traumatic brain injury and persistent symptoms. *Brain Injury* **29**: 688–700.

7. DiFazio M, Silverberg ND, Kirkwood MW, *et al.* (2015) Prolonged activity restriction after concussion: Are we worsening outcomes? *Clin Pediatr (Phila)* [Epub ahead of print].

8. Cantu RC, Gean AD. (2010) Second-impact syndrome and a small subdural hematoma: An uncommon catastrophic result of repetitive head injury with a characteristic imaging appearance. *J Neurotrauma* **27**: 1557–1564.

9. Laskowski RA, Creed JA, Raghupathi R. (2015) Pathophysiology of mild TBI: Implications for altered signaling pathways. In: Kobeissy FH (ed.). *Brain Neurotrauma: Molecular, Neuropsychological, and Rehabilitation Aspects*. Boca Raton, FL.

10. Wang Y, Nelson LD, LaRoche AA, *et al.* (2015) Cerebral blood flow alterations in acute sport-related concussion. *J Neurotrauma* [Epub ahead of print].

11. D'Souza MM, Trivedi R, Singh K, *et al.* (2015) Traumatic brain injury and the post-concussion syndrome: A diffusion tensor tractography study. *Indian J Radiol Imaging* **25**: 404–414.

12. Papa L, Edwards D, Ramia M. (2015) Exploring serum biomarkers for mild traumatic brain injury. In: Kobeissy FH (ed.). *Brain Neurotrauma: Molecular, Neuropsychological, and Rehabilitation Aspects*. Boca Raton, FL.

13. Papa L, Ramia MM, Edwards D, *et al.* (2015) Systematic review of clinical studies examining biomarkers of brain injury in athletes after sports-related concussion. *J Neurotrauma* **32**: 661–673.

14. Papa L, Robertson CS, Wang KK, *et al.* (2015) Biomarkers improve clinical outcome predictors of mortality following non-penetrating severe traumatic brain injury. *Neurocrit Care* **22**: 52–64.

15. Hinson HE, Rowell S, Schreiber M. (2015) Clinical evidence of inflammation driving secondary brain injury: A systematic review. *J Trauma Acute Care Surg* **78**: 184–191.

16. Xiong Y, Peterson PL, Lee CP. (2001) Alterations in cerebral energy metabolism induced by traumatic brain injury. *Neurol Res* **23**: 129–138.

17. Sun X, He G, Qing H, *et al.* (2006) Hypoxia facilitates Alzheimer's disease pathogenesis by up-regulating *BACE1* gene expression. *Proc Natl Acad Sci USA* **103**: 18727–18732.

18. Johnson VE, Stewart JE, Begbie FD, *et al.* (2013) Inflammation and white matter degeneration persist for years after a single traumatic brain injury. *Brain* **136**: 28–42.

19. Johnson VE, Stewart W, Smith DH. (2010) Traumatic brain injury and amyloid-beta pathology: A link to Alzheimer's disease? *Nat Rev Neurosci* **11**: 361–370.

20. Johnson VE, Stewart W, Smith DH. (2013) Axonal pathology in traumatic brain injury. *Exp Neurol* **246**: 35–43.

21. Johnson VE, Stewart W, Smith DH. (2012) Widespread tau and amyloid-beta pathology many years after a single traumatic brain injury in humans. *Brain Pathol* **22**: 142–149.

22. Corsellis JA. (1989) Boxing and the brain. *BMJ* **298**: 105–109.

23. Corsellis JA, Bruton CJ, Freeman-Browne D. (1973) The aftermath of boxing. *Psychol Med* **3**: 270–303.

24. Stein TD, Alvarez VE, McKee AC. (2014) Chronic traumatic encephalopathy: A spectrum of neuropathological changes following repetitive brain trauma in athletes and military personnel. *Alzheimers Res Ther* **6**: 4.

25. Omalu BI, DeKosky ST, Minster RL, *et al.* (2005) Chronic traumatic encephalopathy in a National Football League player. *Neurosurgery* **57**: 128–134; discussion 134.

26. McKee AC, Stern RA, Nowinski CJ, *et al.* (2013) The spectrum of disease in chronic traumatic encephalopathy. *Brain* **136**: 43–64.

27. Stein TD, Alvarez VE, McKee AC. (2015) Concussion in chronic traumatic encephalopathy. *Curr Pain Headache Rep* **19**: 47.

28. Baugh CM, Robbins CA, Stern RA, McKee AC. (2014) Current understanding of chronic traumatic encephalopathy. *Curr Treat Options Neurol* **16**: 306.

29. Petraglia AL, Plog BA, Dayawansa S, *et al.* (2014) The spectrum of neurobehavioral sequelae after repetitive mild traumatic brain injury: A novel

mouse model of chronic traumatic encephalopathy. *J Neurotrauma* **31**: 1211–1224.

30. Petraglia AL, Plog BA, Dayawansa S, *et al.* (2014) The pathophysiology underlying repetitive mild traumatic brain injury in a novel mouse model of chronic traumatic encephalopathy. *Surg Neurol Int* **5**: 184.

31. Turner RC, Lucke-Wold BP, Logsdon AF, *et al.* (2015) The quest to model chronic traumatic encephalopathy: A multiple model and injury paradigm experience. *Front Neurol* **6**: 222.

32. Turner RC, Lucke-Wold BP, Logsdon AF, *et al.* (2015) Modeling chronic traumatic encephalopathy: The way forward for future discovery. *Front Neurol* **6**: 223.

33. Bailes JE, Turner RC, Lucke-Wold BP, *et al.* (2015) Chronic traumatic encephalopathy: Is it real? The relationship between neurotrauma and neurodegeneration. *Neurosurgery* **62**(Suppl. 1): 15–24.

34. McKee AC, Robinson ME. (2014) Military-related traumatic brain injury and neurodegeneration. *Alzheimers Dement* **10**: S242–S253.

35. Goldstein LE, Fisher AM, Tagge CA, *et al.* (2012) Chronic traumatic encephalopathy in blast-exposed military veterans and a blast neurotrauma mouse model. *Sci Trans Med* **4**: 134ra60.

36. Goldstein LE, McKee AC, Stanton PK. (2014) Considerations for animal models of blast-related traumatic brain injury and chronic traumatic encephalopathy. *Alzheimers Res Ther* **6**: 64.

11 What's Going on Now?

"Hope is the bedrock of this nation. The belief that our destiny will not be written for us, but by us, by all those men and women who are not content to settle for the world as it is, who have the courage to remake the world as it should be."

— Iowa Caucus Victory Speech, Barack Obama,
Nobel Laureate (Peace, 2009)

Vitamin E

There are currently five drugs that are Food and Drug Administration (FDA) approved in the USA for the treatment of Alzheimer's disease, but none of them significantly alters the disease process. These drugs and their mechanisms were discussed earlier, and include cholinesterase inhibitors (donepezil, rivastigmine, and galantamine), an N-methyl-D-aspartate (NMDA) receptor) channel blocker (memantine), or a combination of both mechanisms (donepezil and memantine).

In December 2013, *New York Daily News* published a sensational article stating that "the latest hope for slowing [Alzheimer's disease] progression is already on drugstore shelves." The news was based on research at the Mount Sinai's Icahn School of Medicine, showing that vitamin E may delay functional decline by up to 19% per year in people with mild-to-moderate Alzheimer's. This translates into an approximately 6-month benefit over patients who did not take vitamin E. The study found that patients who took a daily 2,000 IU dose of α-tocopherol — the fat-soluble form of vitamin E — were able to maintain activities of daily living such as cooking, shopping, and paying bills at a higher level than those who took a placebo. However, the vitamin E dose did not seem to delay memory loss or cognitive impairment. Another puzzling result was comparing the effects of vitamin E and the FDA-approved Alzheimer's drug memantine. Participants in the study who received both vitamin E and the FDA-approved Alzheimer's drug memantine or memantine alone did not show the same benefits as participants who received vitamin E alone.[1]

This study is encouraging, but it is too early to incorporate high doses of vitamin E into routine Alzheimer's treatment. As per the advice of the Alzheimer's Association, patients should only take vitamin E under the supervision of their physician. Vitamin E, particularly at high doses, can "negatively interact with other antioxidants and medications, including those prescribed to keep blood from clotting or to lower cholesterol."[2]

Medications in the Pipeline

In addition to these current medications (or supplements in the case of vitamin E), there are many other drugs undergoing clinical trials. As discussed in the clinical trial introduction, the path to FDA approval is lengthy, expensive, and stringently regulated. In terms of reaching Phase III clinical trials, nine drug candidates have failed as of spring 2012. The main reason for these failures is a lack of efficacy and toxicity. However, a failed clinical trial does not necessarily mean an end to the science behind the drug. A common thread we see is that the science behind a failed therapy moves forward and is chiseled into a safer or more efficacious solution.

Avenues of new medications fall into two categories: those that try to alleviate the symptoms of Alzheimer's disease and those that aim to stop or delay the disease (usually β-amyloid and/or tau based).

One approach based on β-amyloid clearance or removal from the brain uses anti-β-amyloid antibodies, a special protein that is used by the

Table 11.1.   β-amyloid Immunotherapies in Development (Phases II and III)[3]

Drug class	Drug name	Sponsor	Phase
Monoclonal antibodies	Bapineuzumab	Janssen/Elan/Pfizer	III
	Solanezumab	Eli Lilly	III
	PF-04360365	Pfizer	II
Intravenous immunoglobulin	Gammagard	Baxter/National Institutes of Health	III
	Octagam	Octapharma	II
Active vaccines	CAD106	Novartis	II
	ACC001	Pfizer	II

body's immune system to identify and destroy specific pathogens, or, in this case, β-amyloid (Table 11.1). This approach was realized with the development of a vaccine (AN1792) that was halted in human clinical trials in 2002 due to the occurrence of meningoencephalitis in approximately 6% of patients. Subsequently, several other β-amyloid vaccine immunotherapies have been developed and are under clinical investigation. There are six antibodies in clinical trials using this approach: bapineuzumab (AAB-001) in Phase III, solanezumab (LY2062430) in Phase III, PF-04360365 in Phase II, MABT5102A in Phase I, GSK933776A in Phase I, and gantenerumab (R1450/RO4909832) in Phase I.

Bapineuzumab is targeted to the free amine group at the end of the β-amyloid sequence, or the N-terminus. In a review of the drug, one study writes that Phase II studies of bapineuzumab were "haunted by the ghosts of AN1792."[3] In two trials, approximately 10% of patients who were administered bapineuzumab exhibited vasogenic edema, an accumulation of fluid in the brain that was likely due to disruption of the blood–brain barrier (BBB). The adverse effects of both AN1792 and bapineuzumab both supported a similar theory that particular anti-β-amyloid immunotherapies cause inflammation or other changes in the vessel wall, leading to breakdown of the BBB. The key objective of immunotherapy would thus be to avoid this cause of inflammation while still providing a mechanism of β-amyloid clearance in the brain.

Under the large global American pharmaceutical company Eli Lilly, solanezumab is an antibody that has been developed to target the mid-region of β-amyloid. In small Phase I (19 tested participants) and Phase II (52 participants) studies, there was no evidence of meningoencephalitis (the problem that was found in the first vaccine). Neither was there evidence of vasogenic edema. As the therapy moved forward, however, it showed no therapeutic benefit in two large 18-month Phase III clinical trials in mild-to-moderate Alzheimer's disease patients.[4] Even so, Eli Lilly suggests that there is potential benefit for patients who begin the therapy earlier in the disease progression. In a third trial, the company will extend the two previous trials and give solanezumab to their previously solanezumab-tested patients, as well as to placebo patients. If solanezumab really does provide some therapeutic benefit, there should be a difference between the placebo patients who had a "delayed start" to therapy and so would need to play catch up to the other patients.[5]

Amongst all this talk about β-amyloid, there have been a few studies that focused on tau protein as the primary driver of Alzheimer's disease. In fact, tau pathology correlates better than β-amyloid pathology.[6] Thus, focusing on the clearance of tau aggregates may provide greater clinical efficacy — an area in which we see β-amyloid immunotherapies struggle. At the University of Texas, Galveston, a study by Kayed and colleagues published in the *Journal of Neuroscience* concluded that memory deficits were reversed in Alzheimer's model mice when tau protein was removed. Interestingly, amyloid levels also decreased, suggesting that "tau oligomerization is not only a consequence of [β-amyloid] pathology but also a critical mediator of the toxic effects observed afterward in Alzheimer's disease."[7] This finding went hand in hand with the same research group's discovery of tau oligomer-specific monoclonal antibody (TOMA) just a year earlier. Similar to β-amyloid studies, Kayed and colleagues showed that TOMA could selectively remove the harmful tau in mice, leading to a reversal of memory deficits as well as a reduction in β-amyloid that would naturally accumulate in the Alzheimer's disease state.[8] While efforts to understand the mechanism underlying these β-amyloid antibodies have been ongoing for 16 years, the field of tau immunotherapy is still in its infancy. As of 2016, there are six Phase I clinical trials in this area, while several others are in late-stage pre-clinical development.

Diagnosis

The general consensus regarding Alzheimer's disease treatment is that the earlier a diagnosis can be made, the better it is. Early Alzheimer's disease diagnosis means early action against the chronic degenerative disease. While early treatment may halt or delay symptoms of Alzheimer's, late treatment seems to have "uncertain effects" on the disease.[9] Alzheimer's leaves a mark on the body, a mark that can be observed both physiologically (within the body) and behaviorally (outside the body).

Another term for these physiological changes would be "biological markers," or biomarkers for short, which may indicate that an individual has a certain disease or condition. Although there are currently no proven biomarkers for Alzheimer's, there are several promising candidates that researchers are investigating within the brain, cerebrospinal fluid (CSF), blood, and genome.

Neuroimaging shows great potential for early — perhaps pre-clinical — detection of Alzheimer's disease and for accurately distinguishing the disease in patients with dementias from other etiologies or comorbidities. Computed tomography (CT) and magnetic resonance imaging (MRI) scans, categorically known as structural scans, are used primarily to rule out other conditions that behaviorally look like Alzheimer's but require different treatment (i.e. differential diagnosis) by inspecting the brain's structure. A third important type of brain imaging is positron emission tomography (PET) scan, a technique that makes a three-dimensional image of the functional processes of the body. With PET scans of the brain, researchers and clinicians can see which regions of the brain are less metabolically active due to Alzheimer's — areas related to memory, learning, and problem solving. Contrary to the structural scans, PET scans show the functionality of the brain. These scans use trace amounts of radioactive materials that are injected into a patient's vein prior to imaging. By taking advantage of particular radioactive reagents — such as the Pittsburgh Compound B (PiB) that detects amyloid deposits or fluorodeoxyglucose (FDG) that detects neurodegeneration — clinicians can detect the early onset of Alzheimer's disease and subsequent neurodegeneration due to the disease.[10]

In 2012, the FDA approved the injection of one such radioactive reagent in this area: PiB's longer-lived, fluorodeoxyglucose(F-18)-labeled cousin florbetapir — also known as Amyvid — which was developed by Avid Pharmaceuticals/Eli Lilly and Company.[11] Using Amyvid, clinicians can confidently rule out Alzheimer's with a negative scan. A positive scan, however, does not necessarily mean that a patient has Alzheimer's, since plaques may be present in people with or without Alzheimer's. This got the ball rolling. Two years later, the FDA approved a second amyloid imaging agent: flutemetamol — also known as Vizamyl — which was developed by General Electrics (GE) Healthcare. Vizamyl differs slightly from Amyvid, as it also reports the intensity of amyloid plaques. Experts say that this could make scans easier to read.[12] Neither

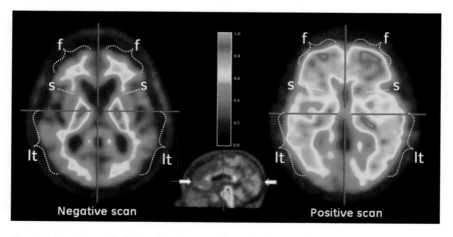

Fig. 11.1. Vizamyl shows the density of amyloid via color images. (Figure credit: Ref. 13.) (f: frontal; s: striatal; lt: lateral temporal.)

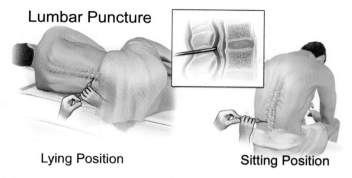

Lumbar Puncture

Lying Position   **Sitting Position**

Fig. 11.2. A lumbar puncture is a minimally invasive procedure for sampling the cerebrospinal fluid (CSF) of a patient. (Figure credit: Ref. 14.)

compound can quantify the amyloid plaques, and this is an area of significant ongoing research.

Remember our discussion of CSF in Chapter 1? CSF surrounds and cushions the brain and spinal cord. The CSF has direct physical contact with the brain and reflects any biochemical changes or toxins that may be building up in the brain. Clinicians take advantage of this by sampling the CSF in a minimally invasive, although potentially painful procedure called a lumbar puncture (LP) (Fig. 11.2).

CSF proteins and metabolites, reflecting the brain's condition, serve as excellent biomarkers of Alzheimer's disease, as well as other neurodegenerative diseases. In Alzheimer's disease, total CSF β-amyloid is not significantly different from controls, but a specific β-amyloid, Aβ42, is comparatively reduced in CSF. Total-tau (t-tau) and phosphorylated tau (p-tau) proteins are both elevated in Alzheimer's disease. Tau is an intracellular protein and p-tau is a component of neurofibrillary tangles (NFTS). This increase suggests neuronal death with the release of tau into the extracellular space.[15] One study compared the extent of these biomarkers in Alzheimer's disease patients and controls. The three biomarkers had good sensitivity, with 90% of Alzheimer's patients being positive for the biomarkers, but poor specificity, as 36% of control subjects were also positive for the biomarkers.[16] This means that biomarkers that are more specific to patients who have Alzheimer's disease alone will be needed in order to better predict who will develop the disease early on. Until then, systematically analyzing both tau and β-amyloid CSF markers may better discriminate Alzheimer's disease than any single marker alone.[17]

Researchers are also investigating whether consistent, measurable changes in blood levels can indicate early, pre-symptomatic Alzheimer's disease. According to the latest research, three interesting metrics are thought to indicate onset of the disease.

At the National Institute on Aging, Kapogiannis and his team gathered blood samples from 70 Alzheimer's patients, 20 diabetic but cognitively healthy elderly patients, and 84 healthy adults. The team identified a single protein from the blood samples, IRS-1 (which is involved in insulin signaling in the brain) to be defective in Alzheimer's patients.[18] A second blood test measures an extensive combination of 10 fats in order to predict dementia with 90% accuracy of clinical onset within 2–3 years. This test was based on blood samples from an astounding 525 people who were aged 70 and older, with the researchers following these individuals as some of them developed memory loss.[19] The study was led by Dr. Howard Federoff and was published in *Nature Medicine* in March 2014. This paper leaves us with hope for Alzheimer's diagnosis, as the biomarker panel that the study found reflected "cell membrane integrity" and may be sensitive enough to detect the early neurodegeneration of pre-symptomatic Alzheimer's disease.[20] A third blood test uses a set of 10 proteins and has 87% accuracy within just a year of dementia onset. Led by Dr. Simon Lovestone, a neuroscience professor at the University of Oxford, this study used blood samples from an astonishing 1,146 subjects who were gathered from three different international studies, consisting of people who had Alzheimer's disease, mild cognitive impairment, or neither. The study concluded that these identified markers may be useful for evaluating disease severity and progression.[21]

An important genetic link that has been implicated in Alzheimer's disease was discovered in 1993. The gene, which is found on chromosome 19, is known as *APOE-e4*. The *APOE-e4* allele is the most studied genetic marker in Alzheimer's disease. The "APOE" part of the gene stands for apolipoprotein-E, which is a normal protein that is integral to cardiovascular health and normal functioning. However, there are several different "versions" (alleles) of the gene, ranging from *APOE-e1* to *APOE-e4*. The *APOE-e4* version of the gene has been implicated in an increased risk of developing Alzheimer's disease (i.e. it is a risk factor); however, it alone does not guarantee the development of the disease, and the absence of the gene does not protect individuals from developing Alzheimer's.

Individuals are able to be screened via genetic testing in order to determine whether or not they carry the *APOE-e4* allele, and if they do, we can gain valuable knowledge about their risk of progressing to Alzheimer's disease in the future. As cited in *The Sports Gene*, "the dementia risk of having a single *Apo-4* gene copy is roughly similar to the risk from playing in the NFL." In particular, having one copy of this gene increases the probability of developing Alzheimer's disease by threefold (8–24%), and having two copies raises the risk to over 75%.[22] As mentioned above, the presence of the allele does not necessary condemn a person to the development of Alzheimer's disease, it simply means that the person is at an increased risk and should work to lower all other risk factors. The utility of understanding what genes contribute to the development of Alzheimer's disease lies in the ability to treat those individuals who are at increased risk before they actually develop any symptoms of cognitive decline. This is known as prophylactic treatment. The only issue currently is that there are no prophylactic treatments available for Alzheimer's disease, but there are many treatments that are being studied. Once an early treatment receives FDA approval, it would be critical to screen individuals, assess their risk of progressing to Alzheimer's disease, and administer the appropriate therapies in order to prevent their decline.

The progress in terms of identifying the genetic risk factors of Alzheimer's disease continues to this day. In 2003, researchers began the National Alzheimer's Disease Genetic Study. This was a federal initiative that sought to collect and store biological samples from patients suffering from Alzheimer's disease, as well as their family members, in order to study and find potential genetic markers that may contribute to the disease process.

As we continue to uncover the genetics behind the development of Alzheimer's disease, we will become better equipped to understand the disease, how to alter its course, how to treat it, and, hopefully, how to prevent it. However, one of the major problems we face when utilizing genomic data in unraveling the disease is simply one of actually finding meaning in the data that we have. Although we have decoded the entire human genome, we are left with a massive amount of data that must be interpreted and understood. The next major project is the Human Proteome Project, which seeks to discover what proteins are encoded by the 23,000 genes in the human genome, and after that, we must come to understand the function of each of these proteins. Thus, genomics is a powerful tool, but also one that amasses huge amounts of data, and finding meaning in these data will likely be the greatest challenge of using genetic information in a clinically meaningful way.

Biomarkers and the Alzheimer's Disease Neuroimaging Initiative Study

The World Wide Alzheimer's Disease Neuroimaging Initiative (WW-ADNI) has been instrumental in the advances that we have made in understanding Alzheimer's disease biomarkers, specifically those related to PET and MRI neuroimaging and changes in blood and CSF. The goals of the WW-ADNI are threefold: (i) to define the rate of progression of Alzheimer's-related cognitive decline; (ii) to develop methods for grouping similar patient populations within Alzheimer's disease; and (iii) to standardize data across all Alzheimer's disease research in order to facilitate collaboration between researchers and clinicians.[23] These three goals culminate into the WW-ADNI's higher objective, which is to gain a comprehensive picture of the impact of Alzheimer's disease across the world.

The ability to predict whether or not a person may develop Alzheimer's disease has tremendous implications not only for an improved understanding of the molecular mechanisms of the disease, but also for the development of interventions. There has been much recent work directed at the establishment of biomarkers and radiological markers of the disease. Tau and amyloid proteins are higher in the CSF of patients with pre-clinical Alzheimer's disease, as well as those with full-fledged Alzheimer's disease.[24,25] The deposition of amyloid proteins is one of the hallmarks of Alzheimer's disease. Amyloid PET is a powerful means of visualizing the *in vivo* deposition of amyloid in the brains of patients using special radioisotopes that can be detected in a noninvasive manner.[26,27] However, the presence of amyloid deposits will not necessarily lead to the clinical signs and symptoms of Alzheimer's disease. The concept of cognitive reserve has been postulated as compensating for the nerve cells that are damaged by amyloid; that is, if there are more neurons, there is greater cognitive reserve.[28]

A concern regarding the above radiological markers and biomarkers of Alzheimer's disease is the considerable overlap between those who have the markers and who develop Alzheimer's disease and those who have the markers but do not develop the disease. There is some prognostic uncertainty that is even greater when one looks at the amyloid and tau levels in the blood.[29] Federoff and colleagues examined exosomes for tau and amyloid levels. Briefly, exosomes are lipid vesicles that are formed within a cell. The neuronal cell makes proteins. Part of the transition and processing of these proteins is via lipid-lined vesicles. Small blebs off of these vesicles result in exosomes, which are extruded out of the cell. The exosomes in Alzheimer's disease patients contain amyloid and tau proteins in higher-than-normal amounts. Exosomes have been postulated to mediate the cell-to-cell spread of pathology by transmitting small bits of protein and nucleic acids (DNA).[30,31] The authors identified patients with Alzheimer's disease who had previously donated blood or blood samples many years before they were diagnosed with Alzheimer's disease. The blood was analyzed and, in particular, the neurally derived blood exosomal levels of phosphorylated tau and β-amyloid proteins were significantly higher in Alzheimer's patients compared to matched control patients. The elevated levels of these biomarkers predated the clinical diagnosis by 1–10 years.

There has been debate as to whether early knowledge of a likely Alzheimer's diagnosis could be detrimental. There certainly are ethical and social consequences of such knowledge. In a study of 63 patients using PET amyloid detection, disclosure of the PET amyloid status did not significantly impact mood or lead to depression. In fact, those subjects with increased amyloid on PET scans were more likely to make positive lifestyle changes (more exercise and a healthier diet) than those with normal amyloid scans.[32]

Studying the Disease

In order to properly study and understand Alzheimer's disease, it is important to have models of the disease. The amount of information that can be acquired from individuals suffering from Alzheimer's disease is limited by technology, the ethics behind putting patients through uncomfortable or invasive procedures in order to collect data or specimens, and the time and resources required in order to effectively conduct clinical studies on patients. One approach to understanding the disease without requiring patients that actually have the disease is by using models — ranging from cells grown in a Petri dish to animals that mimic the pathological processes underlying Alzheimer's disease. These models are extremely useful, as they allow researchers and clinicians to study and understand Alzheimer's disease in a way that would otherwise be unacceptable in humans.

Of the many important contributions that the discovery of these genes led to, one of the most important was the ability to develop models of Alzheimer's disease in mice in order to facilitate the study of the disease process and allow scientists to assay and test new drugs. By understanding the genetic contributions of Alzheimer's disease, such as what genes code for the plaques and tangles found in Alzheimer's brains, in 1995, researchers were able to create mice models that exhibited Alzheimer's pathology and also exhibited the behavioral and cognitive signs found in Alzheimer's. Such mice models are developed by genetically manipulating mice to express the abnormal proteins that are found in Alzheimer's disease, which can then be given drugs, stem cell injections, and other potential therapies that may be thought to alter the trajectory of Alzheimer's disease. The major utility that these mice provide is the ability to study Alzheimer's disease quickly, efficiently, and in a cost-effective manner. Although the mice models are not perfect renderings of Alzheimer's disease in humans, they serve as incredibly important tools. The mice models can be used to screen for drugs that may one day combat Alzheimer's disease in humans. Being able to model a disease is a crucial component to the effective development of ways to treat that disease.

Cells that are grown from patients with Alzheimer's disease can also be cultured in a dish in order to visualize the processes by which the plaques and tangles form and cause disruptions between cells. These cells can come from stem cells that are retrieved from patients themselves or from human embryonic stem cells that can be genetically altered in order to reflect the abnormalities seen in Alzheimer's disease. One revolutionary method in which cells from patients with Alzheimer's disease can be studied is through the creation of induced pluripotent stem cells (iPSCs). Using Dr. Shinya Yamanaka's Nobel Prize-winning work on iPSCs, these "disease-in-a-dish" models can be further personalized since different Alzheimer's patients exhibit different rates of cognitive decline. Thus, the *in vitro* model ("*in vitro*" refers to the study of something outside of a living structure, such as in a Petri dish or flask) can be examined microscopically and serve as an assay of various small molecules, or as a way to better understand the morphological and physiological changes that occur in Alzheimer's disease.

Stem cell models of Alzheimer's disease allow scientists to grow and culture these cells in a Petri dish in order to examine a variety of effects. New experimental drugs, for example, can be added to the cells in order to observe such a drug's effects and toxicity. The cells can be used as a screening tool in order to quickly and efficiently test the myriad of potential new drugs that may influence the underlying pathology of Alzheimer's disease. In addition to drug screening, stem cell models of Alzheimer's disease can be used in order to better understand the pathological changes that occur in Alzheimer's disease. For example, the abnormal proteins that are found in Alzheimer's disease, such as β-amyloid and tau, can potentially be observed and studied in these cell cultures. One limitation, however, is that individual cells in a dish do not adequately reflect the complex environment of cells in living tissue. Therefore, steps are being taken to create more accurate "organ-like" models that can be studied in a dish. For example, in addition to neuronal cells, adding glial cells, vasculature, CSF-producing cells, and immune cells could more accurately replicate the cellular environment of the brain, thus allowing for more accurate models of Alzheimer's disease.

References

1. http://jama.jamanetwork.com/article.aspx?articleid=1810379
2. http://www.alz.org/alzheimers_disease_standard_prescriptions.asp
3. Kerchner GA, Boxer AL. (2010) Bapineuzumab. *Expert Opin Biol Ther* **10**(7): 1121–1130.
4. Doody RS, Thomas RG, Farlow M, *et al.* (2014) Phase 3 trials of solanezumab for mild-to-moderate Alzheimer's disease. *N Engl J Med* **370**(4): 311–321.
5. http://www.nytimes.com/2015/07/23/business/new-data-on-2-alzheimers-drugs-alters-hope-and-expectation.html?_r=1
6. Sigurdsson EM. (2015) Tau immunotherapy. *Neurodegener Dis* **16**(1–2): 34–38.
7. Castillo-Carranza DL, Guerrero-Muñoz MJ, Sengupta U, *et al.* (2015) Tau immunotherapy modulates both pathological tau and upstream amyloid pathology in an Alzheimer's disease mouse model. *J Neurosci* **35**(12): 4857–4868.

8. Castillo-Carranza DL, Sengupta U, Guerrero-Muñoz MJ, *et al.* (2014) Passive immunization with tau oligomer monoclonal antibody reverses tauopathy phenotypes without affecting hyperphosphorylated neurofibrillary tangles. *J Neurosci* **34**(12): 4260–4272.

9. Fagan AM. CSF biomarkers of Alzheimer's disease. *SNM: Advancing Molecular Imaging and Therapy.*

10. http://www.sciencedirect.com/science/article/pii/S0969996114001107

11. http://www.alzforum.org/news/research-news/fda-approves-amyvid-clinical-use

12. http://www.alzforum.org/news/research-news/fda-approves-second-amyloid-imaging-agent

13. http://www3.gehealthcare.com/en/news_center/press_kits/fda_approves_vizamyl

14. https://commons.wikimedia.org/wiki/Category:Lumbar_puncture#/media/File:Blausen_0617_LumbarPuncture.png

15. Aluise CD, Sowell RA, Butterfield DA. (2008) Peptides and proteins in plasma and cerebrospinal fluid as biomarkers for the prediction, diagnosis, and monitoring of therapeutic efficacy of Alzheimer's disease. *Biochim Biophys Acta* **1782**: 549–558.

16. de Meyer G, Shapiro F, Vanderstichele H, *et al.* (2010) Diagnosis-independent Alzheimer disease biomarker signature in cognitively normal elderly people. *Arch Neurol* **67**(8): 949–956.

17. Li G, Sokal I, Quinn JF, *et al.* (2007) CSF tau/Abeta42 ratio for increased risk of mild cognitive impairment: A follow-up study. *Neurology* **69**(7): 631–639.

18. Kapogiannis D, Boxer A, Schwartz JB, *et al.* (2015) Dysfunctionally phosphorylated type 1 insulin receptor substrate in neural-derived blood exosomes of preclinical Alzheimer's disease. *FASEB J* **29**(2): 589–596.

19. http://www.nature.com/news/biomarkers-could-predict-alzheimer-s-before-it-starts-1.14834

20. Mapstone M, Cheema AK, Fiandaca MS, *et al.* (2014) Plasma phospholipids identify antecedent memory impairment in older adults. *Nat Med* **20**(4): 415–418.

21. Hye A, Riddoch-Contreras J, Baird AL, *et al.* (2014) Plasma proteins predict conversion to dementia from prodromal disease. *Alzheimers Dement* **10**(6): 799–807.

22. Topol EJ. *The Patient Will See You Now: The Future of Medicine Is in Your Hands*.

23. http://www.alz.org/research/funding/partnerships/WW-ADNI_overview. asp

24. Rosen C, Hansson O, Blennow K, Zetterberg H. (2013) Fluid biomarkers in Alzheimer's disease — Current concepts. *Mol Neurodegener* **8**: 20.

25. Rosen C, Zetterberg H. (2013) Cerebrospinal fluid biomarkers for pathological processes in Alzheimer's disease. *Curr Opin Psychiatry* **26**: 276–282.

26. Rabinovici GD. (2015) The translational journey of brain beta-amyloid imaging: From positron emission tomography to autopsy to clinic. *JAMA Neurol* **72**: 265–266.

27. Tateno A, Sakayori T, Kawashima Y, *et al.* (2015) Comparison of imaging biomarkers for Alzheimer's disease: Amyloid imaging with [^{18}F]florbetapir positron emission tomography and magnetic resonance imaging voxel-based analysis for entorhinal cortex atrophy. *Int J Geriatr Psychiatry* **30**: 505–513.

28. Bauckneht M, Picco A, Nobili F, Morbelli S. (2015) Amyloid positron emission tomography and cognitive reserve. *World J Radiol* **7**: 475–483.

29. Fiandaca MS, Kapogiannis D, Mapstone M, *et al.* (2015) Identification of preclinical Alzheimer's disease by a profile of pathogenic proteins in neurally derived blood exosomes: A case-control study. *Alzheimers Dement* **11**: 600–607.e1.

30. Rajendran L, Honsho M, Zahn TR, *et al.* (2006) Alzheimer's disease beta-amyloid peptides are released in association with exosomes. *Proc Natl Acad Sci USA* **103**: 11172–11177.

31. Fruhbeis C, Frohlich D, Kramer-Albers EM. (2012) Emerging roles of exosomes in neuron-glia communication. *Front Physiol* **3**: 119.

32. Lim YY, Maruff P, Getter C, Snyder PJ. (2015) Disclosure of positron emission tomography amyloid imaging results: A preliminary study of safety and tolerability. *Alzheimers Dement* [Epub ahead of print].

12 Novel Therapies

Chapter

"Imagination is more important than knowledge. For knowledge is limited, whereas imagination embraces the entire world, stimulating progress, giving birth to evolution. It is, strictly speaking, a real factor in scientific research."

— *Cosmic Religion: With Other Opinions and Aphorisms*
by Albert Einstein, Nobel Laureate (Physics, 1921)

Stem Cells

Stem cells are special cells that have the potential to become any cell in the body. Their power lies in their ability to transform a naïve stem cell into a specific cell type that is normal and healthy and is able to do whatever you want it to do. One of the most promising, yet unsuccessful approaches thus far, for the treatment of Alzheimer's disease is the introduction of stem cells that can secrete protective factors into the brain and help the brain's natural protective mechanisms ward off the disease process. Another approach is actually regenerating the neurons that are lost in Alzheimer's disease, but this approach is fraught with challenges, mainly due to the billions of connections that would need to be remade and the challenges of actually placing the stem cells in the right place at the right time.

One of the oldest and most commonly used stem cell therapies is known as a bone marrow transplant. This is not commonly thought of as a stem cell therapy, but the purpose of the treatment is in essence to replace unhealthy stem cells within the bone marrow of a sick patient with healthy stem cells from a donor. These stem cells are responsible for hematopoiesis, or the development of the various blood cell types within the body. In patients with disorders such as leukemia, the population of bone marrow cells responsible for hematopoiesis are diseased, and by eradicating those cells using radiation and replacing them with healthy cells, the patient's leukemia can be treated. This is the essence of stem cell therapies — replacing damaged cells with healthy cells.

A novel approach to the treatment of Alzheimer's disease using stem cells is to actually increase the production of cerebrospinal fluid (CSF) within the brain. CSF is essentially a fluid that serves many functions — it nourishes and protects the brain, provides essential electrolytes and glucose to the brain, and even clears toxins and the abnormal plaques that accumulate in Alzheimer's disease. Prior research has shown that as people age, the production of CSF decreases. This decrease in CSF production is exacerbated by Alzheimer's disease. One of the authors of this book, Ronald Sahyouni, was fortunate enough to work on a project during medical school at the University of California, Irvine that actually sought to increase the production of CSF in order to treat Alzheimer's disease. The work was being conducted in the laboratory of Dr. Edwin Monuki, a neuropathologist by training and an overall extremely compassionate and motivated mentor who had a personal interest in Alzheimer's disease as well. In his laboratory, induced pluripotent stem cells (iPSCs) were cultured and grown into the ependymal cells that normally create and secrete CSF within the brain. After growing these cells, they were transplanted into the brains of mice in order to see what would happen. It was determined that the cells could actually engraft into the target tissue and reinstate their normal function, which is to secrete CSF[1]. This is a promising potential therapy for Alzheimer's disease, since it would increase the production of CSF, which would nourish and protect the brain using its own endogenous filtration mechanism, and would also decrease the plaque load within the brain, which undoubtedly contributes to the pathological processes of Alzheimer's disease and the destruction of neural connections and cell death.

This is just one example of how neural stem cells can be used in order to potentially treat Alzheimer's disease. Although many of the experimental projects which involve stem cells are still in the earliest phases of research and development, they hold plenty of promise and may one day lead to clinical trials in humans afflicted with Alzheimer's disease and possible cures.

Stem cell transplantation remains a very promising therapeutic approach to the treatment of Alzheimer's disease. By placing cells directly into the brain, the problems of the blood–brain barrier are bypassed. In addition, the cells are able to survive for a prolonged period of time and can work to accomplish their task, whether that be regenerating neural connections, clearing out plaques and tangles, or decreasing the inflammation and increasing the regenerative capacity of the brain. There are several novel approaches that are currently being explored within the field of stem cell transplantations.

Dr. Shinya Yamanaka (along with Dr. John Gurdon) won the 2012 Nobel Prize in Physiology or Medicine for his work on iPSCs. It was due to his work in 2006 that we discovered that a small set of genes could be used to reprogram intact mature cells in mice into immature stem cells. By introducing just four factors, or the Yamanaka factors — Oct3/4, Sox2, c-Myc, and Klf4 — Dr. Yamanaka and colleagues found a way to virtually *turn back the clock*![2] These "disease-in-a-dish" models can be further personalized, since different Alzheimer's patients exhibit different rates of cognitive decline. Thus, the *in vitro* model ("*in vitro*" refers to the study of something outside of a living structure, such as in a Petri dish or flask) can be examined microscopically and can serve as assays for various small molecules, and may even serve as a way to better understand the morphological and physiological changes that occur in Alzheimer's disease.

Lifestyle Modifications

A comprehensive approach to the treatment of Alzheimer's disease includes lifestyle modifications. These modifications must be predicated on research-derived recommendations that have been shown to be neuroprotective against Alzheimer's disease. Lifestyle modifications could include increased sleep time, more cognitive and social activities, and maintaining proper cardiovascular health, to list just a few. Just like in cardiovascular disease, individuals are usually asked by their physician or healthcare provider to do more than just take a medication. They are usually asked to monitor their diet, increase their levels of exercise, avoid certain high-fat and high-cholesterol foods, decrease levels of stress, avoid caffeine, and also monitor their blood pressure, along with many more recommendations. These "lifestyle" modifications extend beyond the prescription pad, allowing individuals to decrease the many risk factors in order to actually prevent or ameliorate heart disease. By changing habits and lifestyle activities, individuals can substantially decrease their risk of developing heart disease.

In 1984, Lee Goldman, MD and MPH and Francis Cook, ScD, from Harvard published a study titled "The Decline in Ischemic Heart Disease Mortality Rates: An Analysis of the Comparative Effects of Medical Interventions and Changes in Lifestyle."[3] They examined all published literature between 1968 and 1976 and estimated that "more than half of the decline in ischemic heart disease mortality ... was related to changes in lifestyle, specifically to reductions in serum cholesterol levels and cigarette smoking. In comparison, about 40% of the decline can be directly attributed to specific medical interventions, with coronary care units and the medical treatment of clinical ischemic heart disease and hypertension being the leading estimated contributors."

These findings reflect the fact that the risk of developing heart disease can be substantially modified by lifestyle modifications. Similarly, lifestyle modifications have been found to directly impact the development of Alzheimer's disease to varying degrees. One important lifestyle modification that has been heavily implicated in the recent literature regarding Alzheimer's disease is sleep. Recently, a new discovery changed our fundamental understanding of the brain. This discovery was predicated on the fact that the brain has no lymphatic system. The rest of the body has an elaborate lymphatic network, which is a loose network of microscopic channels that collect and route excess fluid and debris within tissues to the circulatory system. This lymphatic network acts as a filter for removing excess waste products, fluids, proteins, toxins, and more, bringing them away from tissues and into the bloodstream, where they can then be filtered and removed by the kidneys. It was previously thought that the brain had no lymphatic system. This was proven false in 2015, when two different researchers independently verified the presence of lymphatic vessels within the central nervous system.[4] This was a profound discovery because it changed what was known about the basic building blocks within the brain. The fact that a lymphatic network exists within the brain may allow previously unexplainable phenomenon to be understood, and may even help us to understand more about Alzheimer's disease. This lymphatic system within the brain was coined the "glymphatic" system by Danish neuroscientist Maiken Nedergaard, since the brain's lymphatic system is mediated by glial cells (the supporting cells within the brain).[5] Interestingly, sleep has been found to be an important activity that can actually regulate and modulate how well the glymphatic system works. [The role of sleep and Alzheimer's disease will be discussed in greater detail at the end of Chapter 13.]

A lack of sleep may very well be proportional to the amount of stress a person may experience. Perhaps the lack of sleep leads to greater perceived stress, or maybe stress leads to inability to fall asleep. Either way, a December 2015 study published in the journal *Alzheimer's Disease & Associated Disorders* found that elderly people who regularly feel stressed out have an increased likelihood of developing mild cognitive impairment and thus an increased chance of developing Alzheimer's disease.[6] This idea of individuals feeling stressed is termed "perceived stress" in the literature. "Perceived stress reflects the daily hassles we all experience, as well as the way we appraise and cope with these events," said the study's first author, Mindy Katz, MPH, and senior associate in the Saul R. Korey Department of Neurology at Albert Einstein College of Medicine.[5] Fortunately, perceived stress is a modifiable risk factor for cognitive impairment, and with proactive lifestyle modifications, individuals may be able to lessen the stresses of daily life and decrease their risk of Alzheimer's. Katz mentions some such interventions as including "mindfulness-based stress reduction, cognitive-behavioral therapies and stress-reducing drugs."

Lifestyle modifications and environmental factors can even protect against Alzheimer's disease by increasing the number of connections between neurons in the brain. One of the many environmental factors that can increase the density of synaptic connections within the brain is the degree to which an individual is "linked-in" to their social network. This social network can include anyone from friends, family, colleagues, members of the community, and many more. The reason behind this is that a robust social network engages many different parts of the brain. For example, understanding the relationships between yourself and the various individuals you interact with necessitates the use of multiple circuits within the brain and the formation of new connections as you meet new people. Additionally, being able to converse, interact, and network with the people that you meet requires the global use of the entire brain — in contrast to other tasks such as puzzles, which utilize more discrete networks within the brain.

Studies in which individuals are placed within a functional magnetic resonance imaging scanner and asked to engage in social situations show that the entirety of the brain is activated to a substantial degree in such situations compared to asking that same individual to do specific discrete tasks such as memorizing a list of words. Thus, being connected to a strong social network of friends and family is a beneficial risk modifier when it comes to Alzheimer's disease.[7] Social engagement has been found to improve cognitive health. Mental activities such as reading, watching lectures, playing board games, volunteering, living with someone, and more have been found to improve mental sharpness. A large study of 838 older individuals without dementia found that "higher levels of social engagement in old age is associated with better cognitive function."[8] Specifically, "social activity and social support were related to better cognitive function, whereas social network size was not strongly related to global cognition." These results suggest that the quality of social engagement is more important than the size of your social network.

The Religious Orders Study is a large collaborative study in the United States that involves over 1,100 older religious clergy members, including nuns, priests, and brothers. The study began in 1993 thanks to funding by the National Institute on Aging (NIA), and will continue until June 2016. The participants undergo yearly medical and psychological evaluations and have agreed to donate their brains to science after death. The study is focused on uncovering the changes in the brain that are involved in memory and movement disorders, and also to better understand abnormal declines of cognitive function.[9] This study examined the impact of normal everyday activities such as listening to the radio, reading, and playing games on cognitive health. The results showed that after 4 years of engaging in these activities, the individuals who were the most engaged had a 47% lower risk of developing Alzheimer's disease than the individuals who were least engaged. However, the directionality of this effect is unclear. It is possible that individuals who engaged less frequently in everyday activities such as reading or visiting museums may actually be suffering from the earliest stages of Alzheimer's disease, which could be the reason that they did not engage in activities in the first place. Regardless, it is better to give the results the benefit of the doubt and so engage in social activities and keep your mind mentally engaged, since there are other data that support the protective effects of these actions.

A recent study published in 2010 found that individuals with "lower education had lower cognitive functioning, but this was qualified by level of cognitive activity. For those with lower education, engaging frequently in cognitive activities showed significant compensatory benefits for episodic memory, which has promise for reducing social disparities in cognitive aging."[10] The reason for this may reside in the fact that regular mental activity strengthens the brain circuits involved in learning and memory. Another study published by the same group explored the effects of computer use in males with lower education levels. They found that the use of computers could actually improve mental function.[11] These results strengthen the notion that social engagement and mental activity could improve cognitive health and protect against Alzheimer's disease.

Although social engagement is beneficial, combining a heart-healthy diet and exercise regimen, as well as an intellectually stimulating mental health regimen, has been shown to be even more beneficial.[12] We will discuss the effects of exercise on protecting against Alzheimer's disease later on in the book (see Chapter 13).

Other environmental factors that influence synaptic density and are protective factors against Alzheimer's disease include diet and mental activity. The most current recommendations state that a brain-healthy diet that reduces the risk of heart disease and diabetes and is low in saturated fats and cholesterol can help protect the brain from disease. One study followed 1,409 adults over a period of many years.[13] It found that individuals in the study who were obese in middle age doubled their risk of developing dementia later on in life. Another study examined 8,534 twins from the Swedish Twin Registry and found that midlife obesity and being overweight independently increased the risk of Alzheimer's disease, dementia, and vascular dementia.[14] Even more profound was the finding that individuals with high cholesterol and high blood pressure had a sixfold increase in their risk of developing dementia. These shocking statistics point to the importance that heart- and brain-healthy diets have on the overall development and progression of neurodegenerative and cardiovascular disorders later on in life. Diet plays a crucial role in the development of cardiovascular disease, and a diet that is high in saturated fats and cholesterol increases the chance that arteries throughout the body and brain will become clogged.[15] There are two types of cholesterol: one is known as low-density lipoprotein (LDL) and the other is known as high-density lipoprotein (HDL). LDL is the "bad" cholesterol, and it is best to keep LDL levels as low as possible. This can be achieved by using "healthier" oils such as olive oil, or baking and grilling foods instead of frying food. HDL, on the other hand, is the "healthy" cholesterol, and it is better to have higher levels of HDL compared to LDL. This can be achieved by eating less red meat and more fish, vegetables, and fruits. Although it is not known exactly how much of these foods is needed in order to beneficially contribute to brain health, studies have found that elderly women who ate green, leafy vegetables had a mental age that was 1–2 years younger than women who ate fewer of these vegetables. Cold water fish, such as halibut, tuna, and salmon, are rich in certain fatty acids known as omega-3 fatty acids. These omega-3 fatty acids have been shown to beneficially contribute to cardiovascular health, and thus can also help ward off the development of Alzheimer's disease. Other foods that contain heart-healthy fats include nuts such as almonds, pecans, and walnuts. These nuts also contain vitamin E, which serves as an antioxidant and also helps protect the heart and brain.

Whole grains, red wine, and foods that are rich in antioxidants can also help maintain heart and brain health. One of the more interesting contributions of diet to the avoidance of disease states are from antioxidants. According to the Alzheimer's Association recommendations, dark-skinned fruits and vegetables have the highest levels of antioxidants. These include kale, spinach, broccoli, prunes, raisins, berries, cherries, and more. Antioxidants serve an important role in the body — they effectively neutralize dangerous particles known as free radicals. Free radicals are basically small molecules that are "oxidants," which can attack and damage critical components within the cell. These components can include important proteins or membranes, but most importantly, free radicals can damage DNA. When enough damage has occurred, such a damaged cell can become mutated or killed. This propagates any disease process and weakens the brain's endogenous protective mechanisms. Antioxidants function by neutralizing the free radicals that are floating around in our body. By doing so, they effectively block the potentially damaging effects of these free radicals within the body and bolster the body's ability to ward off damaging disease processes.

One well-known antioxidant that is commonly found in red wine (but also in grapes, berries, and peanuts) is resveratrol.[16] Several studies have sought to explore the protective role of resveratrol in cardiovascular disease and have also found that resveratrol may even help protect individuals from the development of Alzheimer's disease. Studies have found that resveratrol prevents the cleavage of the amyloid precursor protein (APP) in β-amyloid, which forms plaques within the brain. It also serves to enhance the clearance of β-amyloid peptides (which are the abnormal protein aggregates that perpetuate the pathology of Alzheimer's disease) and reduces neuronal damage.[17] Although these outcomes have yet to be proven to prevent or protect against the development of Alzheimer's disease, the addition of heart- and brain-healthy vitamins, antioxidants, phytonutrients, and fats undoubtedly plays some role in the development and progression of the pathology underlying Alzheimer's disease.

Vitamins have also been implicated in lowering the risk of developing Alzheimer's. Certain vitamins, such as vitamin E (an antioxidant) and vitamin C, as well as vitamin B12 and folate, can be protective factors against Alzheimer's. Deficiencies in vitamin B12 can even produce neurological and cognitive symptoms that may resemble Alzheimer's disease. It is critical to maintain a diet that is complete and provides all of the nutrients, vitamins, and minerals that the body needs in order to function properly, but also to balance against taking too much of any one of these vitamins, as some of them in excess can actually be deleterious to one's health. However, diet alone is not enough to effectively protect against Alzheimer's disease. Although diet might delay the onset of Alzheimer's disease, it will not prevent it or significantly alter its course once the disease has manifested itself. Besides diet, exercise is another important environmental factor that can help protect against Alzheimer's.

Exercise is not only critical to heart health due to it lowering the risk of obesity, diabetes, and high blood pressure, but it also helps protect against the chance of developing a stroke, microvascular damage inside the brain, and even a type of dementia known as vascular dementia.

Cardiovascular health is directly linked to brain health, or cerebrovascular health. Since the brain heavily relies on arteries in order to bring blood, oxygen, and nutrients and to remove waste and toxins, having healthy arteries within the brain is crucial. When those arteries are damaged, narrowed due to clogging from fat and cholesterol (known as atherosclerosis), or even blocked completely, the brain is unable to receive the critical support materials that it needs in order to function. This damages the brain, diminishes its ability to defend itself from infections and disease processes, and, if there is enough damage to specific regions of the brain, can even lead to dementia. Exercise reduces the risk of developing various cardiovascular and cerebrovascular diseases. Even when an individual is already suffering from disorders such as high blood pressure, diabetes, or obesity, exercise has been shown to mitigate the harmful effects of these disorders, and can even reverse them to a certain degree.

A healthy exercise regimen also protects against the development of various degenerative disorders later in life, such as vertebral compression fractures, falls, arthritis, and even cartilage degeneration.[18] This can improve an individual's quality of life and increase the likelihood of an individual remaining mentally and physically engaged later on in life, which can ward off the damaging effects of Alzheimer's.

The effect of exercise has been studied in relation to neurogenesis, which is the process of generating new neurons. Neurogenesis is a fairly new concept, as early scientists did not consider the CNS to be capable of regeneration. Its discovery in 1998 by Erikson *et al.* revolutionized neuroscience and brought about exciting new prospects for the treatment of neurological diseases.[19] Research has discovered that exercise stimulates the production of a protein called FNDC5, which is released into the bloodstream.[20] Over time, FNDC5 stimulates the production of another protein in the brain, brain-derived neurotrophic factor (BDNF), which has been found to enhance neurogenesis.[21] Interestingly, the direct infusion of BDNF into animals was not found to reverse Alzheimer's disease pathology, suggesting that other physiological mechanisms may be at play.[22] Additionally, exercise leads to increased blood flow to the brain. This phenomenon has been proven in mouse studies via brain imaging, as well as behavioral studies, in which the mice exhibited a marked increase in neurons and improvements in learning, respectively.[23]

Genetic Modification and Personalized Medicine

Discovered in 2014, the CRISPR/Cas9 system has quickly gain favor within the scientific and medical community as a revolutionary gene editing tool. Taking advantage of the bacterial species *Streptococcus pyogenes*, a group of researchers led by University of California, Berkeley scientists Jennifer Doudna and Emmanuelle Charpetier created the CRISPR/Cas9 system using clustered regularly interspaced short palindromic repeats (CRISPRs), CRISPR associated protein-9 nuclease (Cas9), and hybrid RNA in order to provide an efficient and reliable way to identify, cut, and replace gene sequences.[24] The CRISPR/Cas9 system is relatively easy to use, cheap, fast, and appropriate for germline modification (allowing for a change to be passed from generation to generation). This revolutionary tool has been adopted by researchers in thousands of laboratories in just the 3 years since its discovery.

If gene modification was to be available for human genome engineering, it could be used to eradicate or provide protection from genetic diseases or degeneration. A 2012 study in Iceland suggests that a coding mutation (abbreviated "A673T," which means that an adenine replaced a thymine at the 673rd nucleic acid location in the gene) in the amyloid precursor protein (*APP*) gene protects against Alzheimer's disease and cognitive decline in the elderly without Alzheimer's disease.[25] By targeting the *APP* gene, researchers may be able to significantly decrease the genetic risk factor of Alzheimer's disease by interfering with the production of β-amyloid. Could the CRISPR/Cas9 system then allow us to engineer an *APP* mutation for every newborn, decreasing the genetic risk factor of Alzheimer's disease? Dr. Aubrey de Grey, CEO of the SENS

Research Foundation, takes this a step further and says that the CRISPR system will be central to the delivery of somatic gene therapy in order to combat the aging process, which he views to be a disease, rather than a part of a normal turn of events.

Although the system seems to be the Holy Grail of genetic modification, there is skepticism regarding the biological and social consequences that may come with genetic alteration, in terms of both intended and unintended effects. For example, there is no evidence regarding the unintended consequences of a mutated *APP* gene. Moreover, the ideas of designer babies, modern-day eugenics, and bioterrorism have placed the CRISPER/Cas9 system under scrutiny. It is also unclear if the Food and Drug Administration (FDA) would regulate germline modification if this were to come into the clinic. These are real concerns that have generated substantial controversy. At the 2015 World Stem Cell Summit in Atlanta, Georgia, three experts — Dr. Aubrey de Gray, Dr. Paul Knoepfler and Dr. Aaron Levine — all discussed the huge potential of the system, both positive and negative. Each panelist spoke of different concerns, but there was one unifying thread between all three talks — more voices need to be heard on the topic. Overall, the technology and science is rapidly advancing, but there needs to be dialogue and public policies in order to bring about cures using the CRISPR/Cas9 system in an appropriate, scientifically sound manner.

Low-Level Light Therapy

Revolutionary therapies in photomedicine, a branch of medicine involving the application of light with respect to health and disease, have yielded promising results concerning Alzheimer's disease. Recent studies have shown cognitive and neuronal improvements in mice with early-stage and progressive-stage Alzheimer's disease undergoing low-level laser therapy (LLLT).[26,27] Low-level laser therapy, as the name suggests, refers to the use of single-color lasers at low powers so as not to burn human and animal tissue, but simply to use photostimulation in order to stimulate our body's natural healing processes. Light, whether from the sun or a household lamp, is composed of a collection of colors, some visible and some invisible to the human eye. Each color of light has specific properties associated with it that affect our everyday lives. For example, red, orange, yellow, green, blue, indigo, and violet colors allow us to see the world around us, invisible infrared colors give us heat, and invisible ultraviolet colors can damage our eyes and our skin. The lasers used in low-level laser therapy only use the near-infrared colors of light, which are much less harmful than ultraviolet colors and do not cause cancerous damage to our body. In fact, this specific range of light's colors has been found to have therapeutic effects through their interaction with our body on the microscopic level.

Energy is required in order for animals, including us humans, to survive, grow, and reproduce. We receive this required energy through the digestion of various foods, sugars, and other nutrients by our metabolic processes. These metabolic processes convert the food we consume into chemical energy that can be readily utilized by our body to form new muscle, defend against illnesses, etc. Near-infrared laser light is thought to cause an overall increase in the chemical energy that is obtained from our food by exciting the subcellular structures involved in our metabolic processes of energy production.[28] This increased rate of chemical energy production in an animal's body, including us humans, has been found to increase wound healing with decreased scar tissue formation, to aid in muscle and blood vessel regeneration, to promote hair growth, to decrease symptoms caused by various forms of dementia, and to increase stem cell and immune cell production.[29–36]

One study published in the *Journal of Alzheimer's Disease* in 2011 tested the effectiveness of transcranial LLLT (also known as transcranial laser therapy) for the treatment of mice with early-onset Alzheimer's disease. In this experiment, the researchers non- invasively attached a set of lasers to the shaved scalp (see Fig. 12.1) in a way that yielded an even spread of near-infrared light on the entire outer layer of the brain (cortical layer).

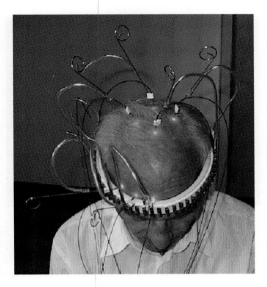

Fig. 12.1.   A typical setup of transcranial laser therapy on a stroke patient. The setup for an Alzheimer's disease patient would be very similar. The lasers are noninvasive and are simply placed on the scalp. (Image obtained from the International Society for Medical Laser Application [ISLA].)

The lasers delivered light either in a pulsed (on-and-off) or continuous manner, and treatment was repeated three times a week for 6 months. After final treatments, the mice were subjected to various cognitive memory tests and found to perform significantly better than mice not treated with transcranial laser therapy. In addition, tissue analysis showed ~30% decreases in β-amyloid proteins for the group treated with a continuous laser and up to 70% decreases in β-amyloid proteins for the group treated with a pulsed laser. The researchers attributed these results to laser-induced increased chemical energy, which caused an increase in neural preservation and a decrease in brain degeneration.

[Another study published in the *Journal of Molecular Neuroscience* in 2015][27] investigated the role of LLLT in mice with progressive-stage Alzheimer's disease by illuminating the bone marrow in order to promote stem cell formation, specifically mesenchymal stem cells that clear

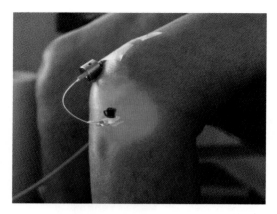

Fig. 12.2.   This is the typical setup for an intra-articular laser therapy that targets the joints instead of the bones. The setup for targeting bone marrow would be identical to this, except the laser would be inserted lower on the leg (tibia) instead of on the knee. (Image obtained from the International Society for Medical Laser Application [ISLA].)

β-amyloid proteins. The team delivered near-infrared laser light to the bone marrow inside of the mouse tibia (the inner bone between the knee and ankle) by invasively placing a fiber optic wire on the surface of the bone (see Fig. 12.2).

This was repeated once every 10 days for a total of six treatments in 2 months. After final treatments, they subjected the mice to various cognitive memory tests and found significantly improved cognitive capacity and spatial learning as compared to mice with progressive-stage Alzheimer's disease not treated with low-level laser therapy. In fact, the performance of the treated Alzheimer's disease mice was almost indistinguishable from that of normal mice. Furthermore, tissue analysis showed increased β-amyloid uptake of 35% within the LLLT treated Alzheimer's disease mice as compared to other non- treated Alzheimer's disease mice. The researchers concluded that these findings suggest an increased immune response and protection against neurodegeneration (brain deterioration).

Although these experiments were carried out in mice, they provide very promising results that could be translated into human trials.

The results suggest that painless and noninvasive low-level laser treatment of the scalp or the slightly painful and invasive low-level laser treatment of the bone marrow could lead to enhancement of the human body's ability to eliminate neurotoxic β-amyloid proteins and increase brain activity in Alzheimer's disease patients, thus slowing or even halting the progression of this mind-crippling disease.

Marijuana (THC)

THC, or Δ9-tetrahydrocannabinol, is a naturally occurring chemical in the marijuana plant. Once consumed, THC binds to cannabinoid (CB) receptors in the brain and affects a person's memory, pleasure, movements, thinking, concentration, coordination, and time perception, according to National Institute on Drug Abuse. THC has been used as an effective medicine for numerous conditions, including glaucoma, epilepsy, asthma, movement disorders, autoimmune diseases, and inflammation, and even to treat psychiatric symptoms in patients with anxiety disorders, sleep disorders, bipolar disorders, and dysthymia.[37]

So, how can this chemical help Alzheimer's disease patients? Well, although THC has not yet been administered to human Alzheimer's disease patients, it has been shown to produce great cognitive improvement in Alzheimer's disease mice and has been proven in the laboratory to inhibit acetylcholinesterase (AChE) more efficiently and with fewer, much milder side effects than the current leading treatments. AChE breaks down a molecule known as acetylcholine. Acetylcholine is an important neurotransmitter (a chemical released by neurons) that is implicated in Alzheimer's disease. Low levels of acetylcholine have been thought to contribute to declines in cognitive function and potentially to play a role in the development of Alzheimer's disease. Therefore, by blocking AChE (the molecule that breaks down acetylcholine), the levels of acetylcholine in the brain can increase. AChE inhibition via THC is done in a way that promotes a higher concentration of brain acetylcholine (which is important for cognition and brain function), while at the same time slowing down the aggregation of β-amyloid proteins (a hallmark pathology of Alzheimer's disease). THC can also reduce neuroinflammation (swelling of the neurons in the brain) and promote the brain's repair mechanisms via the release of BDNFs (factors that guide and assist in the formation of new neurons in the brain). Finally, aside from all of the disease-battling properties of THC, it also induces relaxation and mild euphoria, which may help with the quality of life of the patient as he or she battles this mind-crippling disease.

In a double-blind, 3-year study of donepezil — an AChE inhibitor — researchers discovered that the condition of patients who were taking the drug remained stable for a year or more, but then declined again, although at a rate that was slower than that of the placebo group.[38] This is great news because drugs that slow or halt the progression of Alzheimer's disease — even if only for a little while — are the best treatments currently available to patients. Unfortunately, however, AChE inhibitors, such as donepezil, often have harsh or severe side effects, such as hepatotoxicity (liver damage), nausea, vomiting, loss of appetite, diarrhea, dizziness, muscle cramps, insomnia, and vivid dreams.[39] Here is where THC comes in. THC has superior AChE-inhibiting properties than the leading current treatment (meaning there is a possibility for it to increase cognitive abilities to a higher degree than drugs such as donepezil),[40] while the only side effects it causes are relaxation, sleepiness, mild euphoria, and some undesirable side effects such as decreased short-term memory, dry mouth, impaired perception and motor skills, and red eyes. In new users, THC consumption may cause paranoia or acute psychosis, but these effects are short-lived and their chance of occurrence diminishes as THC usage becomes more regular.[41]

In order to discover the AChE-inhibiting properties of THC, researchers in the Departments of Chemistry, Immunology, Molecular Biology, and Integrated Neurosciences at The Skaggs Institute for Chemical Biology and the Worm Institute for Research and Medicine modeled THC binding to AChE using chemical analysis software. After examining millions of possible scenarios in which these chemicals may interact, they found that THC can bind to two different sites on AChE. THC can bind to the catalytic site of AChE, thus competitively inhibiting it from binding and degrading acetylcholine. When AChE cannot bind to acetylcholine, the brain's acetylcholine levels stay stable, and this is associated with higher cognition in Alzheimer's disease patients. THC can also bind to another region of AChE known as the peripheral anionic binding site (PAS). The PAS is important in Alzheimer's disease because at this binding site, AChE binds to β-amyloid and acts as a molecular chaperone, accelerating the formation of amyloid aggregates.[40] When the PAS is bound to THC, however, it would no longer be able to bind β-amyloid, and this would slow the formation of amyloid plaques. Therefore, this research shows that THC works as a combination of two Alzheimer's disease medications by competitively inhibiting the binding of both acetylcholine and β-amyloid to AChE. This would enhance the patient's cognitive abilities while at the same slowing the aggregation of β-amyloid.

THC and Neurogenesis

Other research into the effects of THC shows that there are numerous CB receptors in the brain, some of which (e.g. CB1 and CB2) become activated upon binding to THC.[42] Interestingly, animal models show that activation of these receptors can increase the production of neurotrophins in the brain.[43] Such findings in animals are a novel discovery, as BDNFs can increase neurogenesis (the production of new neurons) and cognitive performance in Alzheimer's disease mouse models.[44] Evidence of THC's neurogenesis ability was further demonstrated when scientists discovered that mice lacking CB1 receptors showed no adult neurogenesis,[45] and normal mice whose CB receptors were activated with a synthetic CB showed higher neurogenesis than controls.[46] Because the culprit behind the decline in the cognitive abilities of Alzheimer's disease patients is neurodegeneration (death of neurons) and synaptic loss, these findings are very important in terms of treatment. With increased levels of BDNF (a protein that promotes survival and plasticity in neurons) and increased neurogenesis, Alzheimer's disease patients might be able to recover some of their lost cognitive abilities, as well as experience a delay in the progression of Alzheimer's disease.

THC and Inflammation

When accumulation of amyloid plaques in the brain starts to cause synaptic loss and neuronal death, the body naturally responds by prompting the microglial cells in the brain to produce pro-inflammatory molecules to attack whatever is causing the problem. This unfortunately ends up backfiring, and these pro-inflammatory molecules also end up causing even more neuronal death. THC reduced this neuroinflammation by activating and upregulating (increasing the number of) CB2 receptors of microglial cells in the regions where amyloid plaques are present.[47,48] This activation of CB2 receptors causes microglial cells in the brain to produce fewer pro-inflammatory molecules and more anti-inflammatory molecules.[49,50] This means that THC can significantly decrease inflammation in the areas that are being affected most by the build-up of amyloid plaques, thus giving brain cells a greater chance of survival — possibly even increasing the patient's cognitive function.

Alzheimer's disease remains a devastating neurodegenerative disorder for which no cure exists. Current treatments for Alzheimer's disease are mostly unsuccessful, and even if they slow the progression of the disease for a short time — as cholinesterase inhibitors do — it is at the cost of severe side effects such as liver toxicity (hepatotoxicity) and abdominal (gastrointestinal) disturbances. For this reason, the active compound in cannabis (THC) should be considered as an alternative and more efficacious treatment for Alzheimer's disease. By activating the CB pathways in the brain, THC stimulates the release of BDNF, which increases neurogenesis and thus battles the Alzheimer's disease-induced neurodegeneration head on. It can bind to AChE and competitively inhibit it from binding to acetylcholine or β-amyloid, thereby increasing the brain's concentration of acetylcholine and decreasing the rate at which amyloid plaques form. It can decrease neuroinflammation, thus giving brain cells a higher chance of survival. It has very mild side effects when compared to other drugs that have been approved for Alzheimer's disease, and it can even serve as a palliative treatment for the depression caused by Alzheimer's disease by inducing relaxation and mild euphoria in the user. With time, THC could become a potentially useful tool in the comprehensive treatment of Alzheimer's; however, the safety and efficacy of THC use in Alzheimer's patients must be further studied. Other, less controversial alternative therapies have also been studied, and one such approach is music therapy.

Music Therapy

The current treatment for Alzheimer's disease is best described as a multi-targeted approach because it is actually a combination of treatments that differ greatly in their nature. They vary from chemically synthesized pharmaceuticals to help from social workers, nursing homes, and family members. These treatments either aim to battle the different pathologies of the disease or serve as palliative treatments in order to reduce the anxiety, stress, anger, and depression that are caused by it. One interesting treatment in this multi-targeted approach is called music therapy. Music therapy is the use of music by a music therapist in order to address the physical, emotional, cognitive, or social needs of a patient. It involves creating, singing, moving to, and/or listening to music that corresponds to the weaknesses, strengths, and preferences of the patient. Music therapy also provides avenues for communication that can be helpful to patients who find it difficult to express themselves in words.[51]

Music therapy is grouped into two fundamental methods: the receptive method — which is listening based — and the active method — which is based on the patient's participation in playing, singing, or dancing to music.[51] Current research has shown that both methods can be significantly effective palliative therapies in the multi-targeted treatment of Alzheimer's disease. The receptive method can aid Alzheimer's patients by helping them recall and connect with events from their long-term memory and by significantly reducing the anxiety and stress caused by their illness. The active method has been proven to decrease the behavioral and psychiatric symptoms of the disease — which include delusions, agitation, apathy, irritability, aberrant movements, and nighttime disturbances.[52] As a result, the combination of these two methods of music therapy holds tremendous benefit for Alzheimer's patients. This is especially true because current alternative treatments that reduce anxiety, depression, and psychiatric symptoms involve chemically synthesized pharmaceuticals such as neuroleptics, sedatives, and antidepressants, which have adverse side effects and complications.

In a study published in 2009 in the journal *Dementia and Geriatric Cognitive Disorders*, researchers discovered significant improvements in anxiety and depression in Alzheimer's patients who participated in receptive music therapy for 16 weeks. They also noted that the reduction in stress and anxiety was sustained for at least 8 weeks after the discontinuation of therapy sessions. These researchers enrolled patients living in the Les Violettes nursing home, who all suffered from mild-to-moderate Alzheimer's, in a randomized controlled study. They separated the 30 study participants into two groups: 15 in the music therapy group and 15 in the control group. Over the course of the next 16 weeks, they administered receptive music therapy sessions once a week to the music therapy group while administering different sessions to the control group that consisted of reading a book and resting. The music chosen for the music therapy sessions was based on each patient's personal tastes and preferences and was played in the patient's room as the patient rested in a comfortable chair or bed. Each session lasted approximately 20 minutes.[52] The researchers clinically evaluated all 30 participants at weeks 4, 8, 16, and 24, which was 8 weeks after the final session. They observed significant improvements in anxiety (Fig. 12.3) and depression (Fig. 12.4) in the patients in the music therapy group as compared to the control group, and saw that these decreases in anxiety and depression persisted even after the therapy had been stopped for 8 weeks.

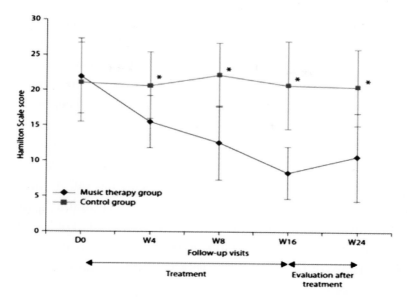

Fig. 12.3. The Hamilton Scale score is a measure of anxiety. Receptive music therapy significantly lowers anxiety and maintains low anxiety at up to 8 weeks after treatment. (Figure credit: Ref. 51.)

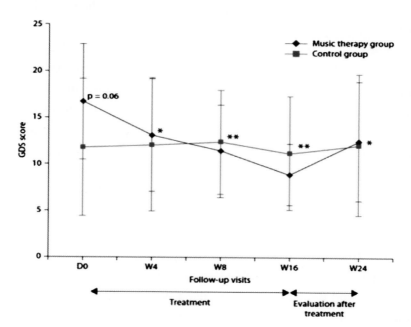

Fig. 12.4. The Geriatric Depression Scale (GDS) score is a measure of depression. Receptive music therapy significantly lowers depression and maintains low depression at up to 8 weeks after treatment. (Figure credit: Ref. 51.)

The sessions also seemed to help stimulate cognitive function by encouraging memory encoding and recall. Patients were recorded claiming, "This music reminds me of my childhood and my family," or "I pictured myself at the ball, dancing how we used to," or "This reminds me of my journeys with my husband."[51] This suggests that receptive music therapy improves autonomy in patients suffering from Alzheimer's disease by evoking autobiographical events and stimulating memory recall.

Another study published in 2008 in the journal *Alzheimer's Disease and Associated Disorders*[52] highlighted the effects of music therapy — this time the active method — on the behavioral and psychiatric symptoms of Alzheimer's disease. This study consisted of 59 patients with moderate-to-severe dementia, of whom 48 (81%) had Alzheimer's disease. Thirty of the 59 patients were selected for the music therapy group and 29 were selected for the control group. The music therapy group participated in 30 sessions of active music therapy, with each session being 30 minutes long. During these sessions, the patients were encouraged to smile, sing, or dance with the music. The control group, however, participated in educational and entertainment activities such as reading a newspaper, playing cards, personal care, lunching, bathing, etc. All patients were clinically evaluated before treatment, 8 weeks into treatment, 16 weeks into treatment, and 4 weeks after the end of the 16-week treatment period. The results from the cognitive assessment of these patients showed significant reductions in delusions, agitation, anxiety, apathy, irritability, aberrant movements, and nighttime behavioral disturbances for those in the music therapy group as compared to those in the control group. This reduction in behavioral and psychiatric symptoms persisted for up to a month after the end of treatment.[53]

In closing, whether receptive or active, music therapy is a great palliative treatment for the symptoms of Alzheimer's disease. This natural, noninvasive, and enjoyable therapy can significantly decrease anxiety, stress, and the behavioral/psychiatric symptoms of dementia. It has no side effects, which is especially beneficial if we consider that the only alternative treatments for the same symptoms cause severe adverse side effects and complications. Finally, it encourages cognitive stimulation by allowing patients to recall and connect with their past memories and may thus allow patients to stimulate, use, and discover their remaining memories or abilities. Music therapy fits perfectly into a multi-targeted approach for the treatment of Alzheimer's disease.

References

1. Lehtiner *et al.* (2013). *J Neurusg* 33 (45): 17553–17554.
2. Takahashi K, Yamanaka S. (2006) Induction of pluripotent stem cells from mouse embryonic and adult fibroblast cultures by defined factors. *Cell* **126**(4): 663–676.
3. Goldman L, Cook EF. (1984) The decline in ischemic heart disease mortality rates: An analysis of the comparative effects of medical interventions and changes in lifestyle. *Ann Intern Med* **101**(6): 825–836.
4. Dissing-Olesen L, Hong S, Stevens B. (2015) New brain lymphatic vessels drain old concepts. *EBioMedicine* **2**(8): 776–777.
5. https://en.wikipedia.org/wiki/Glymphatic_system
6. http://www.newswise.com/articles/stress-in-older-people-increases-risk-for-pre-alzheimer-s-condition
7. http://www.alz.org/we_can_help_remain_socially_active.asp
8. Krueger KR, Wilson RS, Kamenetsky JM, *et al.* (2009) Social engagement and cognitive function in old age. *Exp Aging Res* **35**(1): 45–60.
9. https://www.rush.edu/services-treatments/alzheimers-disease-center/religious-orders-study
10. Lachman ME, Agrigoroaei S, Murphy C, Tun PA. (2010) Frequent cognitive activity compensates for education differences in episodic memory. *Am J Geriatr Psychiatry* **18**(1): 4–10.
11. Tun PA, Lachman ME. (2010) The association between computer use and cognition across adulthood: Use it so you won't lose it? *Psychol Aging* **25**(3): 560–568.
12. Wang H-X, Karp A, Winblad B, Fratiglioni L, *et al.* (2002) Late-life engagement in social and leisure activities is associated with a decreased risk of dementia: A longitudinal study from the Kungsholmen project. *Am J Epidemiol* **155**(12): 1081–1087.

13. Kivipelto M, Ngandu T, Laatikainen T, *et al.* (2006) Risk score for the prediction of dementia risk in 20 years among middle aged people: a longitudinal, population-based study. *Lancet Neurol* **5**(9): 735–741.

14. Xu WL, Atti AR, Gatz M, *et al.* (2011) Midlife overweight and obesity increase late-life dementia risk: A population-based twin study. *Neurology* **76**(18): 1568–1574.

15. http://www.alz.org/we_can_help_adopt_a_brain_healthy_diet.asp

16. Li F, Gong Q, Dong H, Shi J. *et al.* (2012) Resveratrol, a neuroprotective supplement for Alzheimer's disease. *Curr Pharm Des* **18**(1): 27–33.

17. Ma T, Tan MS, Yu JT, Tan L, (2014) Resveratrol as a therapeutic agent for Alzheimer's disease. *Biomed Res Int* 2014: 350516.

18. Otterness IG, Eskra JD, Bliven ML, *et al.* (1998) Exercise protects against articular cartilage degeneration in the hamster. *Arthritis Rheum* **41**(11): 2068–2076.

19. Eriksson PS, Perfilieva E, Björk-Eriksson T, *et al.* (1998) Neurogenesis in the adult human hippocampus. *Nat Med* **4**(11): 1313–1317.

20. Huh JY, Panagiotou G, Mougios V, *et al.* (2012) FNDC5 and irisin in humans: I. Predictors of circulating concentrations in serum and plasma and II. mRNA expression and circulating concentrations in response to weight loss and exercise. *Metabolism* **61**(12): 1725–1738.

21. Binder DK, Scharfman HE. (2004) Mini review. *Growth Factors* **22**(3): 123–131.

22. Budni J, Bellettini-Santos T, Mina F, *et al.* (2015) The involvement of BDNF, NGF and GDNF in aging and Alzheimer's disease. *Aging Dis* **6**(5): 331–341.

23. van Praag H, Shubert T, Zhao C, Gage FH. (2005) Exercise enhances learning and hippocampal neurogenesis in aged mice. *J Neurosci* **25**(38): 8680–8685.

24. Jinek M, Chylinski K, Fonfara I, *et al.* (2012) A programmable dual-RNA-guided DNA endonuclease in adaptive bacterial immunity. *Science* **337**(6096): 816–821.

25. Jonsson T, Atwal JK, Steinberg S, *et al.* (2012) A mutation in APP protects against Alzheimer's disease and age-related cognitive decline. *Nature* **488**(7409): 96–99.

26. de Taboada L, Yu J, El-Amouri S, *et al.* (2011) Transcranial laser therapy attenuates amyloid-β peptide neuropathology in amyloid-β protein precursor transgenic mice. *J Alzheimers Dis* **23**(3): 521–535.

27. Farfara D, Tuby H, Trudler D, *et al.* (2015) Low-level laser therapy ameliorates disease progression in a mouse model of Alzheimer's disease. *J Mol Neurosci* **55**(2): 430–436.

28. Karu T. (2007) *Ten Lectures on Basic Science of Laser Phototherapy.* Gragesberg,Sweden: Prima Books.

29. Bibikova A, Belkin V, Oron U. (1994) Enhancement of angiogenesis in regenerating gastrocnemius muscle of the toad (*Bufo viridis*) by low-energy laser irradiation. *Anat Embryol (Berl)* **190**(6): 597–602.

30. Bibikova A, Oron U. (1993) Promotion of muscle regeneration in the toad (*Bufo viridis*) gastrocnemius muscle by low-energy laser irradiation. *Anat Rec* **235**(3): 374–380.

31. Shefer G, Oron U, Irintchev A, *et al.* (2001) Skeletal muscle cell activation by low-energy laser irradiation: A role for the MAPK/ERK pathway. *J Cell Physiol* **187**(1): 73–80.

32. Shefer G, Partridge TA, Heslop L, *et al.* (2002) Low-energy laser irradiation promotes the survival and cell cycle entry of skeletal muscle satellite cells. *J Cell Sci* **115**(Pt 7): 1461–1469.

33. Oron U, Yaakobi T, Oron A, *et al.* (2001) Attenuation of infarct size in rats and dogs after myocardial infarction by low-energy laser irradiation. *Lasers Surg Med* **28**(3): 204–211.

34. Oron U. (2011) Light therapy and stem cells: A therapeutic intervention of the future. *Interv Cardiol* **3**(6): 627–629.

35. Tuby H, Maltz L, Oron U. (2011) Induction of autologous mesenchymal stem cells in the bone marrow by low-level laser therapy has profound beneficial effects on the infarcted rat heart. *Lasers Surg Med* **43**(5): 401–409.

36. Tuby H, Hertzberg E, Maltz L, Oron U. (2013) Long-term safety of low level laser therapy at different power densities and single or multiple applications to the bone marrow in mice. *Photomed Laser Surg* **31**(6): 269–273.

37. cannabis-med.Org

38. Winblad B, Wimo A, Engedal K, *et al.* (2006) 3-year study of donepezil therapy in Alzheimer's disease: Effects of early and continuous therapy. *Dement Geriatr Cogn Disord* **21**(5–6): 353–363.

39. Querfurth HW, LaFerla FM. (2010) Mechanisms of disease. *N Engl J Med* **362**(4): 329–344.

40. Eubanks LM, Rogers CJ, Beuscher AE 4th, *et al.* A molecular link between the active component of marijuana and Alzheimer's disease pathology. *Mol Pharm* **3**(6): 773–777.

41. NLM: National Library of Medicine. (2006) Marijuana intoxication: MedlinePlus Medical Encyclopedia. [https://www.nlm.nih.gov/medlineplus/ency/article/000952.htm] [Accessed December 3, 2015].

42. Piomelli D. (2003) The molecular logic of endocannabinoid signalling. *Nat Rev Neurosci* **4**(11): 873–884.

43. Galve-Roperh I, Aguado T, Palazuelos J, Guzmán M. (2007) The endocannabinoid system and neurogenesis in health and disease. *Neuroscientist* **13**(2): 109–114.

44. Lee J, Duan W, Long JM, *et al.* (2000) Dietary restriction increases the number of newly generated neural cells, and induces BDNF expression, in the dentate gyrus of rats. *J Mol Neurosci* **15**(2): 99–108.

45. Jin K, Peel AL, Mao XO, *et al.* (2004) Increased hippocampal neurogenesis in Alzheimer's disease. *Proc Natl Acad Sci USA* **101**(1): 343–347.

46. Kim SH, Won SJ, Mao XO, *et al.* (2006) Role for neuronal nitric-oxide synthase in cannabinoid-induced neurogenesis. *J Pharmacol Exp Ther* **319**(1): 150–154.

47. Benito, C, *et al.*, (2003) "Cannabinoid CB2 receptors and fatty acid amide hydrolase are selectively overexpressed in neuritic plaque-associated glia in Alzheimer's disease brains." *Neurosci.* **23**(5): 11136–11141.

48. Ramírez BG, Núñez E, Tolón RM, *et al.* (2005) Prevention of Alzheimer's disease pathology by cannabinoids: Neuroprotection mediated by blockade of microglial activation. *J Neurosci* **25**(8): 1904–1913.

49. Facchinetti F, del Giudice E, Furegato S, *et al.* (2003) Cannabinoids ablate release of TNFα in rat microglial cells stimulated with lypopolysaccharide. *Glia* **41**(2): 161–168.

50. Molina-Holgado F, Pinteaux E, Moore JD, *et al.* (2003) Endogenous interleukin-1 receptor antagonist mediates anti-inflammatory and neuro-protective actions of cannabinoids in neurons and glia. *J Neurosci* **23**(16): 6470–6474.

51. http://www.musictherapy.org/about/musictherapy/

52. Guétin S, Portet F, Picot MC, *et al.* (2009) Effect of music therapy on anxiety and depression in patients with Alzheimer's type dementia: Randomised, controlled study. *Dement Geriatr Cogn Disord* **28**(1): 36–46.

53. Raglio A, Bellelli G, Traficante D, *et al.* (2008) Efficacy of music therapy in the treatment of behavioral and psychiatric symptoms of dementia. *Alzheimer Dis Assoc Disord* **22**(2): 158–162.

13 How Can We Solve the Problem?

"We cannot solve our problems with the same thinking we used when we created them."

— Albert Einstein, Nobel Laureate (Physics, 1921)

In order to adequately address the problem of Alzheimer's disease, we must attack it on several fronts, just like in cardiovascular disease, in which if an individual is at risk of developing a heart attack, they are given many tools to ward off this possibility. One of the most important tools that has lessened the burden of cardiovascular disease on our population has been early screening measures such as blood test-derived biological markers, or biomarkers. Before biomarkers were utilized, an individual's risk was mainly determined by their family history, blood pressure, lipid profile, and other clinical signs or symptomatic manifestations of cardiovascular disease. This allowed doctors to estimate an individual's risk of developing cardiovascular disease. However, this was not enough. Before the discovery of the first cardiac biomarkers in 1954,[1] the morbidity and mortality of cardiovascular disease was higher simply because the disease could not be detected until late into its progression. However, we must at the same time keep in mind that before the advent of fast food and widely prevalent sedentary lifestyles, individuals generally were at a lower risk of developing cardiovascular disease than they are now.

After the discovery of biomarkers, physicians became able to simply order a blood test and screen for various markers of early disease.

This allowed doctors to accurately stratify patients according to their risk of developing disease. Those at higher risk could be started on risk-reduction therapies such as medications, weight loss, exercise programs, and lifestyle modifications. This helped prevent the aggressive onset of cardiovascular disease and allowed individuals to live longer, healthier, and more productive lives.

Early detection, early intervention, appropriate medications and therapies, and comprehensive lifestyle medications have drastically reduced the morbidity and mortality of individuals who follow their treatment regimens. This comprehensive approach to the treatment of a disease is an ideal way of staving off the deleterious consequences of cardiovascular disease, and a similar approach must be taken for Alzheimer's disease.

Caregiving

We have previously discussed just how deleterious Alzheimer's disease is, not only on the patient, but on the family and caregivers. In addition to helping patients with informal care, caregivers may be confidants, surrogate decision makers, and advocates for the patient. This can be draining to so many facets of a caregiver's life. One way to measure the burden of caregiving is financially. In 2009, nearly 11 million Americans provided unpaid care that totaled 12.5 billion hours to family members and friends with Alzheimer's disease. This is equivalent to $144 billion.[2] Something much more difficult to quantify is the emotional strain that is being added on top of the financial and physical stresses. In a state of chronic stress and exhaustion, caregivers are more likely to neglect their own health, more likely to smoke and consume saturated fats, and less compliant regarding their own medication management.[3]

Many caregivers and loved ones of afflicted individuals selflessly dedicate their lives to making sure that their loved ones are well taken care of and supported during the course of their disease. This is not only extremely demanding on the part of the caregiver, but can also lead to significant amounts of psychological stress, suboptimal lifestyle changes, and negative impacts on the caregiver's livelihood, career, family life, and more. It is imperative that individuals who are caring for loved ones who are afflicted with any medical condition ensure that they take care of themselves mentally and physically. This is particularly crucial in disorders such as Alzheimer's disease, which last many months or years. It is relatively manageable to temporarily disrupt one's lifestyle in order to care for an acutely ill individual, as is the case when a family member or loved one is injured or has the flu. However, in diseases that require long-term management and care of loved ones, it is exponentially more difficult for the caregiver to adjust their lifestyle in order to provide care.

One of the caregiving options for patients with Alzheimer's disease is Alzheimer's-specific caregiving centers. These centers are usually privately owned facilities that specialize in providing care to individuals with dementia and Alzheimer's disease. These centers can help families care for their loved ones with Alzheimer's disease in a feasible way, and offer an alternative to standard in-home caregiving by family members or hired healthcare professionals.

The comprehensive management of Alzheimer's disease requires some component of ensuring that the family and loved ones caring for the individual with Alzheimer's also remember to care for themselves. This can be achieved by educating the family and loved ones regarding the possible dangers of not taking care of themselves as well. The potential for depression, anxiety, burning out, extreme stress, physical conditions that could be triggered by a sedentary lifestyle, and even financial disarray for caregivers are all real problems that need to be considered and avoided when possible. Consistent reminders by the patient's physician or healthcare provider to the family and caregivers should be provided, in addition to potentially screening caregivers for signs of depression, stress, anxiety, and burning out. The ultimate goal is to provide patients and their families with as much support and knowledge and as many resources as possible in order to ensure that their only responsibility is taking care of themselves and spending as much quality time as possible with their loved ones who are afflicted with Alzheimer's.

Comprehensive and Integrative Care Clinics

In the future treatment of Alzheimer's disease, it would be ideal to have specialized clinics across the country that are focused on the holistic management of patients suffering from the disease, and also patients who may be at risk of developing the disease. These clinics would specialize in risk stratification, risk reduction and management, early diagnosis, prophylactic treatment, and lifestyle modifications that have been shown to play a neuroprotective role in Alzheimer's disease. These factors will be discussed in the following sections.

Risk Stratification

One of the first steps that should be taken when beginning the management of a patient who is older than 50 years of age should be a comprehensive evaluation of that patient's risk of developing dementia, specifically Alzheimer's disease. This risk evaluation can include a comprehensive family history, a baseline neuropsychological assessment, positron emission tomography scan (either glucose or Pittsburgh compound B (PiB)) (see Figs. 13.1 and 13.2),[4] cardiovascular and cerebrovascular risk factor assessment, and, eventually, the implementation of any biomarkers that may be developed to screen for the development of Alzheimer's disease. Based on the results of this comprehensive risk evaluation, patients can be placed on different observation protocols, which would include repeat measurements of their cognitive functions at discrete intervals in order to detect subtle changes in cognitive capacity that may be indicative of the development of Alzheimer's disease.

Understanding a patient's risk is a critical component of eventually eradicating Alzheimer's disease. Patients with the highest risk could be

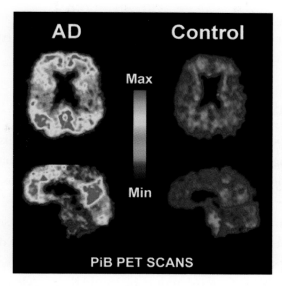

Fig. 13.1. The Pittsburgh Compound B (PiB) PET scan can image amyloid deposits in the brain. Higher levels of amyloid show increased uptake of PiB in Alzheimer's disease patients (left) compared to normal brains. (Figure credit: Ref. 5.)

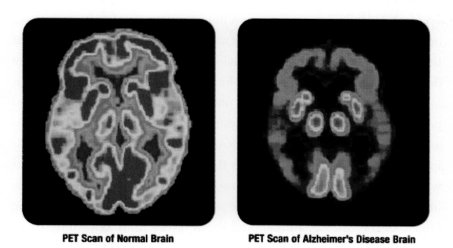

Fig. 13.2. A PET scan that uses radiolabeled glucose shows that the brains of patients with Alzheimer's disease (right) utilize glucose less effectively than normal brains (left). Glucose uptake is a marker of normal brain function. (Figure credit: Ref. 6.)

followed closely and initiated on therapies and lifestyle modifications early in order to thwart the onset of disease. This is the first step in the comprehensive management of Alzheimer's disease.

Risk Reduction and Management

Another important step in preventing the onset of disease would be attempting to reduce the risk factors that a patient may have. For example, if the patient has cardiovascular disease, which has been shown to contribute to the development of Alzheimer's disease, appropriate steps can be taken in order to treat the underlying cardiovascular disease and therefore decrease that risk factor's contribution to the development of Alzheimer's disease.

Another example of risk reduction would be lifestyle modifications. A sedentary lifestyle that is intellectually dry may exacerbate the pathology of Alzheimer's disease — this risk factor can be modified by creating an exercise regimen that the patient can ascribe to, as well as encouraging the patient to be involved in cognitively stimulating tasks, such as taking classes in person or online, engaging in social interactions, or finding an intellectually stimulating hobby. Research has shown that the more socially affluent an individual, the lower their likelihood of developing Alzheimer's disease. This may be because of the fact that interacting with friends and family encourages the use of many different parts of the brain, and when the brain is being used frequently, there is an increase in the density of synaptic connections between neurons. This increase in synaptic density means that there are stronger connections within the brain, and as any disease process begins to deteriorate the integrity of the connections, there is more resilience to the damaging effects of the disease. In addition, social interactions and exercise can increase synaptic density, as was discussed previously. Interestingly, mutations in synaptic proteins have been found to be associated with autism, which is a neurodevelopmental disorder resulting in varying degrees of impairment in social interactions. When the mutation found in families with autism was placed into mice, researchers found impaired social interactions in the mice.[7] The degree to which social interactivity in humans is correlated to synaptic density is variable; however, according to the National Institute on Aging (NIA), social engagement is associated with a lower risk of Alzheimer's disease.[8]

There is a saying that "neurons that fire together, wire together." This statement effectively conveys the notion that whenever various neurons and neural circuits within the brain are activated at the same time, they are prone to developing connections with one another. Thus, activities that cause the entire brain or many different neural circuits to be activated at once will increase the likelihood that new connections will be formed. This is exactly what is desired in order to increase synaptic density and resist against disease processes that destroy connections between neurons.

Risk reduction would potentially delay the clinical manifestations of Alzheimer's disease, and any delay in the onset of the disease is crucial for a variety of reasons. Firstly, the social impact of Alzheimer's disease would be mitigated, as the patient and their loved ones would be able to spend more time together. This means that there is less stress related to caring for a loved one who is afflicted with Alzheimer's, less economic burden nationally due to less time away from work as loved ones care for their family members, more time to enjoy friends and family in one's elder years, and a dramatic decrease in mortality related to Alzheimer's disease. If the onset of Alzheimer's disease could be pushed back by only 5 years, the prevalence of the disease would decrease by 40% by 2035.[9] The reason for this is that there are many other diseases that an individual would be more likely to develop if Alzheimer's disease did not affect that individual, and thus the cause of death would not be due to Alzheimer's disease, but rather another less cognitively devastating disorder.

Early (Correct) Diagnosis

Once risk stratification has been completed, there still exists a further very important step in the comprehensive management of a patient with

Alzheimer's disease: correct diagnosis of the disease. One of the major issues with Alzheimer's disease is that its diagnosis is quite complex. There are many other neurological disorders that may mimic the symptoms of Alzheimer's, especially early on. These include dementia with Lewy bodies, frontotemporal dementia, vascular dementia, and many other causes of dementia that must be considered before giving someone a diagnosis of Alzheimer's disease. Although Alzheimer's is the most common cause of dementia, it is certainly not the only one. Alzheimer's disease has a completely different pathophysiological process that underlies the cognitive changes that eventually lead to dementia compared to other causes of dementia. It is imperative that the appropriate diagnosis is made.

One of the ways in which a clinical diagnosis of Alzheimer's disease is made after a comprehensive neuropsychological assessment, which includes hours of tests, a clinical history and neurological examination, and usually imaging and laboratory tests, all evaluated by an appropriately trained neurologist. Patients are often diagnosed with Alzheimer's disease without going through appropriate testing measures, and thus live for many years with an incorrect diagnosis.

Prophylactic Treatment

The ideal way to treat any disease is to delay its onset as much as possible. Thus, the term "prophylactic" refers to treatment that is meant to prevent the onset of symptoms, and thus delay the progression of the disease. For example, an individual with an elevated risk of developing a heart attack could be given a medication regimen consisting of lipid-lowering agents and blood thinners such as aspirin. These medications are meant to prevent the formation of a blood clot that would block one of the arteries within the heart and thus lead to a heart attack. Prophylactic treatment is crucial to effectively decreasing the prevalence of any disease, yet one issue with prophylactic treatments for Alzheimer's disease is that none exists.

In order to effectively combat Alzheimer's disease, a multifaceted approach towards the treatment and prevention of the disease must be implemented. Once an individual is appropriately diagnosed with Alzheimer's disease, a comprehensive treatment regimen must be instituted. This regimen should consist of a realistic exercise regimen, improved sleep hygiene, lifestyle modifications in order to alleviate the memory problems associated with Alzheimer's, and the institution of appropriate medication therapy. Although there are only a handful of drugs that provide clinically minute improvements in the progression of Alzheimer's disease, they should be considered in the comprehensive treatment of a patient who is newly diagnosed with Alzheimer's disease. The ideal scenario in the future would be the early appointment of medications that are even better than what currently exists today. Unfortunately, most medications lead to only minor improvements in patients who are afflicted with Alzheimer's disease, so patients would greatly benefit from better medications.

Diet

As part of a comprehensive approach to the treatment of Alzheimer's disease, lifestyle modifications must be addressed. The six pillars of a brain-healthy lifestyle consist of exercise, a healthy diet, cognitive stimulation, proper sleep, healthy levels of stress, and an active social life. Some have suggested that inflammation and insulin resistance (as seen in diabetes) can contribute to neuronal injury and alter healthy synaptic communication between neurons, implicating metabolic disorders such as diabetes with disturbances in neuronal function and communication. One aspect of lifestyle is diet. Current evidence suggests that a diet that is rich in fruits, vegetables, and whole grains and low in sugar and saturated fats can protect the brain.

Two diets that have been specifically studied and are believed to be beneficial to cardiovascular and neuronal health are the Dietary Approaches to Stop Hypertension (DASH) and the Mediterranean-DASH

Intervention for Neurodegenerative Delay (MIND). In addition, ginger, green tea, fish, soy, and berries can help protect cells, especially glial cells within the brain, from damage. Glial cells help maintain a healthy brain and remove toxins from the brain — protecting glia is an important component of protecting the brain. Additionally, avoiding trans-fats and saturated fats (sometimes referred to as partially hydrogenated oils) is important, since these can lead to the formation of free radicals, which are molecules that can damage cells. Fatty dairy products, red meat, fast and fried food, and processed foods are rich in trans-fats and saturated fats and should be avoided. Instead of trans-fats and saturated fats, healthy omega-3 fats should be consumed. The docosahexaenoic acid (DHA) found in omega-3 fatty acids (which come from cold-water fish, including salmon, and fish oil supplements) can be neuroprotective and can help reduce the plaque load within the brain. Green tea has also been suggested to improve memory and cognition, likely due to the neuroprotective effects of the antioxidants found in green tea, which neutralize free radicals within the brain.[10]

The DASH diet recommends fruits, vegetables, low-fat dairy items, whole grains, fish, chicken, nuts and beans, vegetable oils, low sodium and sugar intake, and reduced red meat consumption. The MIND diet similarly recommends reduced red meat consumption, whole grains, fruits and vegetables, fish, nuts, and olive oil.[11]

In a study in which participants underwent annual neurological evaluations from 1997 through the Rush Memory and Aging Project at Rush University in Chicago, 923 adults with an average age of 80 years and without Alzheimer's disease at the start of the study were followed. They had to complete questionnaires regarding their diet between 2004 and 2013. The study suggested that the MIND diet can decrease the risk of Alzheimer's disease by 53% amongst individuals who strictly adhere to the diet, and by 35% for those who adhered to it consistently well. The author of the study commented that "even moderate adherence to the MIND diet showed a statistically significant decreased risk of developing Alzheimer's disease ... [and] neither the Mediterranean diet or DASH had that benefit with moderate adherence." The MIND diet recommends at least three servings of whole grains daily, six servings of leafy green vegetables weekly in addition to one additional vegetable daily, bi-weekly servings of berries, weekly servings of fish, bi-weekly servings of poultry, three servings of legumes (e.g. beans) weekly, five servings of nuts weekly, and a daily serving of alcohol (ideally red wine). Olive oil is also recommended as the primary oil to be used in cooking, and the diet recommends reducing red meat consumption, fast or fried food consumption, and sweet consumption to less than five times a week, and little use of butter or margarine. The DASH and Mediterranean diets were also shown to reduce the risk of Alzheimer's disease. However, only in individuals who strictly adhered to these diets were the results significant. The DASH diet reduced the risk by 39%, while the Mediterranean diet reduced the risk by 54%. Fruits are emphasized in both diets, and berries in particular are recommended due to their antioxidant content.[12]

In addition to a normal healthy diet, some supplements such as folic acid, vitamin B12, vitamin D, magnesium, and fish oil can help protect the brain. These nutrients can readily be obtained from a healthy diet; however, in diets lacking essential healthy nutrients such as vitamin B12 or magnesium, supplements can be beneficial. Vitamin E, ginkgo biloba, coenzyme Q10 and turmeric have also been suggested to help with Alzheimer's disease[12]; however, the data are less supportive for these supplements. Ideally, these nutrients should come from food instead of supplements, and supplements containing iron, aluminum, or copper should be avoided when possible, as they may be harmful in excess.[13]

One recent study[14] explored the polyphenols found in pomegranates, which have been reported to have neuroprotective effects, especially in Alzheimer's disease, in transgenic animal models. However, the exact molecule that could be behind these neuroprotective effects was unknown. It is known that pomegranates are rich in a class of polyphenols known as ellagitannins, specifically punicalagin, which is hydrolyzed and transformed into ellagic acid (EA) within the body. EA is transformed by bacteria in the gut into urolithins, which can enter the body and are found to have neuroprotective and anti-inflammatory effects. The study attempted to unravel the mystery behind the beneficial compound from pomegranate extract. The same group that published the study had previously found that pomegranate extract protects against Alzheimer's disease in animals models. In this study, they used computational models in order to predict what compounds could permeate and break through the blood–brain barrier (BBB), and it was found that one pomegranate extract molecule, known as a urolithin, was able to penetrate the BBB. Urolithins were found by the group to prevent the formation of β-amyloid, and could potentially play a role in protection against Alzheimer's disease.

References

1. Dolci A, Panteghini M. (2006) The exciting story of cardiac biomarkers: From retrospective detection to gold diagnostic standard for acute myocardial infarction and more. *Clin Chim Acta* **369**(2): 179–187.
2. https://www.alz.org/national/documents/report_alzfactsfigures2009.pdf
3. Navaie-Waliser M, Feldman PH, Gould DA, *et al.* (2002) When the caregiver needs care: The plight of vulnerable caregivers. *Am J Public Health* **92**(3), 409–413.
4. https://commons.wikimedia.org/wiki/File:PET_scan-normal_brain-alzheimers_disease_brain.PNG
5. https://commons.wikimedia.org/wiki/File:PiB_PET_Images_AD.jpg
6. https://commons.wikimedia.org/wiki/File:PET_scan-normal_brain-alzheimers_diesease_brain.png
7. Hines RM, Wu L, Hines DJ, *et al.* (2008) Synaptic imbalance, stereotypies, and impaired social interactions in mice with altered neuroligin 2 expression. *J Neurosci* **28**(24): 6055–6067.
8. https://www.nia.nih.gov/alzheimers/publication/preventing-alzheimers-disease/search-alzheimers-prevention-strategies
9. https://www.alz.org/documents_custom/trajectory.pdf

10. http://www.helpguide.org/articles/alzheimers-dementia/alzheimers-and-dementia-prevention.htm

11. http://www.alz.org/research/science/alzheimers_prevention_and_risk.asp#exercise

12. http://www.prevention.com/health/diet-lowers-alzheimers-risk

13. http://www.pcrm.org/health/reports/dietary-guidelines-for-alzheimers-prevention

14. http://pubs.acs.org/stoken/presspac/presspac/full/10.1021/acschemneuro.5b00260

14 What Resources Exist?

"A fellow who does things that count, doesn't usually stop to count them."

— Albert Einstein, Nobel Laureate (Physics, 1921)

Although change occurs quite slowly in the scientific world, it seems as if change occurs even more slowly in the political world. Unfortunately, there is an interesting dichotomous link between science and politics. Science relies on the funding programs that are governed by political bodies, yet it wants to be relatively independent from political influences in terms of what is being studied and how it is being studied. Science, ranging from basic science to clinical research, undoubtedly benefits society. It is within the public interest to promote and encourage scientific discovery from economic, humanitarian, and public health standpoints. Fortunately, there are several government, non-profit, and for-profit programs that seek to further the goals of Alzheimer's disease research, ranging from groundbreaking discoveries made in the laboratory to bringing the latest therapies to patients at the bedside.

In order to garner political support to pass and fund the bills and proposals that are put on the table by legislators, lobbying is an unfortunate reality of furthering the cause of Alzheimer's disease.

The national government, specifically the National Institute on Aging (NIA) — a branch of the National Institutes of Health (NIH) — recognizes the public health impact of Alzheimer's disease. The NIA was created by Congress in 1974 to facilitate research, training, and the generation of educational programs pertaining to aging and seniors. Future amendments eventually designated the NIA as the primary federal agency of Alzheimer's disease research. The National Institute of Neurological Disorders and Stroke (NINDS) also supports basic and translational research related to Alzheimer's disease by funding major medical institutions across the country. The NIA and NINDS, along with several more important organizations such as the US Department of Veterans Affairs, the National Science Foundation, and the US Department of Defense, come together to track the Alzheimer's disease fight and update the National Alzheimer's Plan accordingly. This plan includes research and funding strategies, the supervision of translational research from bench to bedside, and reports of ongoing clinical trials. The fact that there are so many organizations working towards one unifying goal — finding effective curative and preventative measures against Alzheimer's disease — highlights the importance of the mission.

Global Resources

According to the Alzheimer's Association, Alzheimer's disease effects 47 million people worldwide and costs $604 billion per year, and it projects that 76 million individuals will have Alzheimer's disease by 2030 and 131.5 million by 2050.[1,2] Sadly, an individual is diagnosed with dementia every 4 seconds, and this incidence is on the rise. In a global poll, 59% of individuals around the world believed Alzheimer's disease to be a normal part of aging. Furthermore, 40% of the individuals surveyed believe that Alzheimer's disease is not fatal, and 37% of individuals believe that a family history of Alzheimer's disease is required in order to be at risk of developing it. Interestingly, Alzheimer's disease comes in as the second most "feared" disease or condition, at 23% (second to cancer at 42%). A total of 96% of individuals who were surveyed also felt that being self-sufficient throughout their lives is very important, and 71% of individuals believe that the government is responsible for helping to find a cure for Alzheimer's disease.[3]

The United Nations (UN) developed a Non-Communicable Disease Political Declaration in 2011. Non-communicable diseases (NCDs) refer to diseases that cannot be "transmitted" from person-to-person, including heart disease, cancer, and Alzheimer's disease. The declaration called for countries to develop NCD prevention plans and NCD research and to mitigate the development of NCDs. So far, 22 countries around the world have developed a "national plan" that is focused on Alzheimer's disease and dementia. The plans are meant to create a blueprint of the impact of Alzheimer's disease and dementia in the country, and list a series of objectives for addressing the impact of Alzheimer's disease. The implementation of these national plans also makes the country more accountable for their successes or failures in addressing dementia, and allows the country to monitor their progress towards ameliorating the impact of Alzheimer's disease. The creation and implementation of these plans began in 2004 with Australia, followed in 2006 by South Korea, in 2007 by Norway, in 2008 by France and The Netherlands, in 2009 by England, in 2010 by Denmark and Scotland, and in 2011 by Northern Ireland and Wales. After these countries drafted national plans with discrete objectives towards eradicating Alzheimer's disease, Finland, the USA, and Japan followed suit in 2012, followed by Israel, Luxembourg, Switzerland, and Taiwan in 2013, Costa Rica, Cuba, Mexico, and Italy in 2014, and Malta in 2015. These countries, and many more, have also become part of Alzheimer's Disease International (ADI), which is an international federation of Alzheimer's groups that was created by the Alzheimer's Association. The ADI focuses on increasing awareness of dementia and lobbying for policy change at the national level and in accordance with the World Health Organization (WHO). In 2012, the WHO released a publication entitled *Dementia: A Public Health Priority*, which called for international awareness of dementia, research, and quality of life improvements for individuals suffering from dementia. The WHO actually had its first Ministerial Conference on Global Action against Dementia in March of 2015. This conference was held in Geneva, Switzerland, and had representatives from 89 countries, who spent several days sharing plans on how to address dementia. This led to the creation of a WHO-mandated Call for Action, which encourages member nations to advocate for dementia awareness and to focus on early diagnostic measures, dementia research, and support groups for individuals with dementia and their caregivers.

Following this conference, in October of 2015, the WHO regional office for North and South America, called the Pan-American Health Organization (PAHO), created the first comprehensive strategic plan focused on dementia. This plan, entitled *Strategy and Plan of Action on Dementia in Older Persons*, specifically focuses on enhancing the quality of life and caregiving resources for individuals with dementia, and calls for mitigating cognitive decline and improving dementia research. As mentioned previously, the G8 Summit on Dementia held in London, England, similarly focused on addressing dementia and identifying a cure or treatment for Alzheimer's disease by 2025. Furthermore, the G8 Summit hoped to improve funding for dementia research, improve data and research sharing on an international level, and create a focused plan of action in order to facilitate dementia research. This led to a worldwide response, with countries such as England, Canada, Japan, and the USA creating new collaborations and models for enhancing research funding, research collaboration, caregiving support, and the dissemination of research progress on an international level. The G8 Summit also created the World Dementia Council, which focuses on coordinating Alzheimer's research on a global level. The council is composed of 19 members from a variety of backgrounds (public health officers, scientists, economists, advocates, etc), and is working to coordinate a global response against Alzheimer's disease.

In March of 2015, a prospectus by the Global Alzheimer's Platform (GAP) composed of the New York Academy of Sciences and the Global CEO initiative GCEOi on Alzheimer's Disease was released. The prospectus focused on integrating international efforts on Alzheimer's disease in order to create a global clinical trial platform focused on reducing the clinical trial cycle time and enhancing clinical

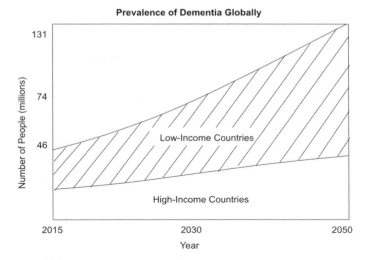

Fig. 14.1. The increase in the prevalence of dementia around the world is shown. Specifically, dementia is expected to disproportionately impact lower-income countries around the world. (Modified from Ref. 52.)

trial efficiency and uniformity. The goal of the GAP is to provide better proof-of-concept trials that could help bring therapies to patients more quickly.[4] The GAP prospectus reflects the diverse range of efforts that are being employed in order to curb the effects of Alzheimer's disease. At a personal, industrial, business, national, and international level, individuals around the world are coming together in order to address the problems of Alzheimer's disease and dementia. However, without determination and an unwavering commitment to action, these efforts could easily go unnoticed and must be continually infused with support at all levels.

Federal Resources (Lobbying) to Fund Alzheimer's Research Programs and Scientists

Lobbying is advocacy activity directed towards influencing a legislator's vote on a particular decision. The legislator can be an individual up to an entire government entity.

This fight has united families and politicians alike. In 2013, Representative Erik Paulsen, a Republican representing the Twin Cities western suburbs, and Representative Keith Ellison, a Democrat representing Minneapolis, engaged in a bipartisan public discussion on Alzheimer's disease. The congressmen set aside differences and focused on the shared objective in order to overcome the Alzheimer's disease epidemic. These two individuals are members of the Alzheimer's Association Young Champions, a diverse group of emerging community leaders who are dedicated to changing the face of Alzheimer's disease and related dementias by raising awareness across generations.[6] As Young Champions, these leaders represented the Alzheimer's Association in order to lobby for more funding towards research and discovery for addressing Alzheimer's disease. However, you do not have to be congressman to join the fight.

On another level, advocates in the Alzheimer's Association — one of the largest advocacy and support group for Alzheimer's disease — are active year-round, engaging elected officials within all aspects of the government. The annual Alzheimer's Association Advocacy Forum in Washington, DC, brings together hundreds of such advocates from throughout the United States in order to understand the current state of the disease and to meet members of Congress so as to lobby for Alzheimer's legislative priorities.

Just as disparate as the legislator to whom an individual may lobby, there may also be differences in how to lobby. Advocacy for Alzheimer's disease can come in the form of writing — opinion pieces on Community Voices at Congress — to asking for more funding or education — explaining of the Alzheimer's fight to others.

Organizational and Support Groups for Families

Many medical diagnoses are extraordinarily difficult to comprehend, digest, and deal with. Some of the more devastating diseases, such as cancer or dementia, can leave patients and their families feeling extremely vulnerable or worried, and they usually necessitate a vast amount of resources and support from friends and organizations. Receiving care and support extends beyond the doors of a hospital room or doctor's office. The patient must live with the disease and needs to receive care in a holistic and comprehensive manner. One of the most useful avenues for the dissemination of information is from support groups and forums in which patients and their families can hear from and ask questions of other individuals who are afflicted with similar diseases. A support group helps patients and their families find some comfort by learning that other individuals are able to live and deal with a devastating condition, and these groups can offer some solace and hope to patients and their families. Support groups for patients with Alzheimer's disease and their caregivers exist online and in person. A simple Google search with the terms "Alzheimer's support group" yields a plethora of links to groups that can and should be integrated into the comprehensive plan of care for a patient with Alzheimer's disease. The Alzheimer's Association[7] even has a specialized website that is tailored to helping caregivers and patients find support groups in their area. These groups provide an intimate forum in which individuals can provide tips, guidance, and advice and share their own personal struggles and triumphs with others. Sometimes, the recommendations made by fellow patients and caregivers outweigh the recommendations that come from busy clinicians who may not have the time or first-hand experience of dealing and struggling with a particular disease as other patients or caregivers. The added value of these groups can eventually lead to the incorporation of attending weekly or monthly support groups into the lifestyle of Alzheimer's patients, and could serve as an avenue for stress relief or grieving for the patients and their families. In the process, such patients and families may provide invaluable support and advice to other local families. These moments of high stress, even hopelessness may serve to establish lasting bonds.

Ultimately, the comprehensive approach to the treatment of Alzheimer's is crucial. From the discovery of new treatments, understanding of the pathological and cellular processes that may underlie the disease, and finding better ways to diagnose and care for patients with Alzheimer's disease, every step is critical in the fight against Alzheimer's. Finding the empathy to relate to a patient with Alzheimer's disease is simple enough, but finding the motivation to become an activist, to speak out for promoting awareness and understanding of the disease, and even trying to work to support the abolishment of Alzheimer's can be a struggle. The daily lives of most individuals is jam-packed and busy, so finding the time not only to understand, but also to create genuine change in the world can be challenging. However, whether it is Alzheimer's disease, diabetes, or cancer, it is critical to create change first hand. Where we stand in the world of medicine today is due to the millions of changes created by our predecessors. As Sir Isaac Newton once said, "If I have seen further it is by standing on the shoulders of Giants."[8] Individuals who have a desire to take ideas and translate them into actionable events and forge meaning from the sculpture of time may walk away from life with a newfound understanding of the power of the human condition.

Inaction is a difficult activity when an individual has seen the power of change and witnessed science and medical breakthroughs treat incurable diseases. HIV was once an incurable disease that lead inevitably to AIDS. However, to the surprise of many, HIV has transformed from an incurable disorder to a disease that can be chronically managed, and individuals with HIV can actually live long and normal lives. In fact, the HIV/AIDS fight is seen as a success story — of patients, scientists, regulatory agencies, and governments coming together and expediting the path towards treatment. The hope is that the same can be said about Alzheimer's — that one day, people will look back and applaud the interdisciplinary forces that came together to combat the disease.

Change is bound to come, although at times it is painfully slow. We have to accelerate our fight because lives are on the line. Change comes from the ideas, will, and action of individuals around the world who have set attainable objectives in order to accomplish a goal. Oliver Wendell Holmes Sr. stated that "every now and then a man's mind is stretched by a new idea or sensation, and never shrinks back to its former dimensions." For many individuals, this "new idea" is a cure for Alzheimer's disease. Once that idea has been visualized, it is difficult not to work towards realizing that idea. As a homage to those who have lost their lives in the fight and to support the endeavors of the scientists, researchers, businessmen and women, national leaders, and those who are at risk, the fight to treat and cure Alzheimer's disease must not be attenuated. Rather, the fight should be reinvigorated continuously. Given the cutting-edge breakthroughs that are occurring and novel approaches to understanding and changing the course of Alzheimer's disease, there are many opportunities for offering current and prospective patients an alternative course of treatment that will work, improve quality of life and change the course of the disease. Ellen Johnson Sirleaf, Nobel Laureate (Peace, 2011), said that "future generations will judge us not by what we say, but what we do." We urge anyone who has picked up this book to continue on their path of education, outreach, and advocacy, so that they can contribute to future generations and hopefully make this book obsolete.

References

1. https://alz.org/global/
2. http://www.alz.org/advocacy/global-efforts.asp
3. https://alz.org/global/InternationalSurvey.pdf
4. http://www.usagainstalzheimers.org/sites/default/files/pdfs/gap_march_2015.pdf
5. http://www.alz.org/advocacy/global-effects.asp/
6. http://www.alz.org/mnnd/in_my_community_22308.asp
7. http://www.alz.org/apps/we_can_help/support_groups.asp
8. http://digitallibrary.hsp.org/index.php/Detail/Object/Show/object_id/9285

Acknowledgements

The authors of this book would like to acknowledge and thank the many individuals who helped us in the research, creation, and completion of this book. The guidance, assistance, and support of our friends, families, and colleagues was invaluable throughout the duration of this project. Specifically, we would like to acknowledge the following individuals for their direct contributions and assistance in the creation and preparation of this book:

Amin Mahmoodi (content contributor)

Amir Mahmoodi (content contributor)

Geri McClure (editing and feedback)

Magdalena Paszkowska (content contributor)

Note to Readers

We intend that in reading this book, you have gained valuable insight into Alzheimer's disease and the human brain. In order to enhance awareness, we hope that you will take proactive steps to educating and informing your friends, family members, and loved ones regarding Alzheimer's disease. In addition, we would like to ask you to share your constructive comments and thoughts regarding this book by reviewing it online. A constructive review of this book on Amazon.com or any online review forum would be much appreciated by the authors of this book, and will also help educate and inform future readers.

Glossary/Abbreviations

Preface

AIDS	Acquired immune deficiency syndrome
FDA	Food and Drug Administration
HIV	Human immunudeficiency virus
MD	Medical doctor
NIA	National Institute on Aging

Chapter 1

CAT	Computed axial tomography
CNS	Central nervous system
CSF	Cerebrospinal fluid
CT	Computed tomography
Dura	Protective covering around the brain
ED	Emergency department
Glia	Support cells in the brain
H.M.	Famous patient who had his hippocampus removed
MRI	Magnetic resonance imaging
Myelin	Fatty wrapping around brain cells
Neuron	Brain cell

Chapter 2

CNS	Central nervous system
FOXO3	Forkhead box O3

LV	Lateral ventricles
OB	Olfactory bulb
PNS	Peripheral nervous system
Presbyopia	Stiffening of the lens in the eye
RMS	Rostral migratory stream
SGZ	Subgranular Zone
SVZ	Subventricular Zone
Telomeres	Protective "ends" of chromosomes
TBI	Traumatic brain injury

Chapter 4

APP	Amyloid precursor protein
cSDH	Chronic subdural hematoma
CTE	Chronic traumatic encephalopathy
CUMC	Columbia University Medical Center
ER	Endoplasmic reticulum
mRNA	Messenger RNA
NPH	Normal pressure hydrocephalus
NYSPI	New York State Psychiatric Institute
PD	Parkinson's disease
TBI	Traumatic brain injury
UPR	Unfolded protein response

Chapter 5

Aβ42	β-amyloid 42
APOE	Apolipoprotein E (gene implicated in Alzheimer's disease)
APP	Amyloid precursor protein
CSF	Cerebrospinal fluid
CT	Computed tomography
DLB	Dementia with Lewy bodies
MRI	Magnetic resonance imaging
NIH	National Institutes of Health

NIMH	National Institute of Mental Health
PD	Parkinson's disease
PET	Positron emission tomography
SPECT	Single-photon emission computed tomography

Chapter 6

ADI	Alzheimer's Disease International
BDNF	Brain-derived neurotrophic factor
CDC	Centers for Disease Control and Prevention
GAAIN	Global Alzheimer's Association Interactive Network
HRT	Hormone-replacement therapy
IADRP	International Alzheimer's Disease Research Portfolio
MCI	Mild cognitive impairment
NAPA	National Alzheimer's Project Act
NIA	National Institute on Aging
NIH	National Institutes of Health
SNP	Single-nucleotide polymorphism
WHIMS	Women's Health Initiative Memory Study
WHO	World Health Organization

Chapter 7

AN1792	β-amyloid vaccine
CAD106	β-amyloid vaccine
CHIs	Cholinesterase inhibitors
DIAN	Dominantly Inherited Alzheimer's Network
FDA	Food and Drug Administration
NHS	National Health Service
NICE	National Institute for Health and Care Excellence
NMDA	N-methyl-D-aspartate
PET	Positron emission tomography
PiB	Pittburgh Compund B
QLs	Quantity limits

Chapter 8

APP	Amyloid precursor protein
CSF	Cerebrospinal fluid
EQ	Encephalization quotient
Homo sapiens	Human species
PSEN1	Presenilin 1 (gene implicated in Alzheimer's disease)
PSEN2	Presenilin 2 (gene implicated in Alzheimer's disease)

Chapter 9

CSF	Cerebrospinal fluid
DBS	Deep-brain stimulation
FDA	Food and Drug Administation
iPSCs	Induced pluripotent stem cells

Chapter 11

APOE-e4	Genetic allele associated with Alzheimer's disease
CSF	Cerebrospinal fluid
FDA	Food and Drug Administration
iPSCs	Induced pluripotent stem cells
MRI	Magnetic resonance imaging
PET	Positron emission tomography
PiB	Pittsburgh Compound B
t-tau	Total tau
p-tau	Phosphorylated tau
TOMA	Tau oligomer-specific monoclonal antibody
WW-ADNI	World Wide Alzheimer's Disease Neuroimaging Initiative

Chapter 12

A673T	Adenine replaced a thymine at the 673rd nucleic acid location
AChE	Acetylcholinesterase

APP	Amyloid precursor protein
BDNF	Brain-derived neurotrophic factor
Cas9	CRISPER-associated protein-9 nuclease
CB	Cannabinoid
c-Myc	Factor implicated in stem cells
CRISPRs	Clustered regularly interspaced short palindromic repeats
CSF	Cerebrospinal fluid
FDA	Food and Drug Administration
Gastrointestinal	Abdominal
GDS	Geriatric Depression Scale
Hepatotoxicity	Liver toxicity
HDL	High-density lipoprotein
In vitro	Studies not done in animals
In vivo	Studies done in animals
iPSCs	Induced pluripotent stem cells
ISLA	International Society for Medical Laser Application
Klf4	Factor implicated in stem cells
LDL	Low-density lipoprotein
Oct3/4	Factor implicated in stem cells
PAS	Peripheral anionic binding site
Sox2	Factor implicated in stem cells
THC	Δ9-tetrahydrocannabinol or marijuana

Chapter 13

BBB	Blood–brain barrier
DASH	Dietary Approaches to Stop Hypertension
EA	Ellagic acid
Glucose	Sugar
MIND	Mediterranean-DASH Intervention for Neurodegenerative Delay
NIA	National Institute on Aging

| PET | Positron emission tomography |
| PiB | Pittburgh Compound B |

Chapter 14

ADI	Alzheimer's Disease International
DoD	US Department of Defense
GAP	Global Alzheimer's Platform
NCDs	Non-communicable diseases
NIA	National Institute on Aging
NIH	National Institutes of Health
NINDS	National Institute of Neurological Disorders and Stroke
NSF	National Science Foundation
PAHO	Pan-American Health Organization
UN	United Nations
VA	US Department of Veterans Affairs
WHO	World Health Organization

Index

Alois Alzheimer, 121–123
Alzheimer's, 49–56
Alzheimer's Association, 236, 237, 240, 241
Alzheimer's disease biomarkers, 184
Alzheimer's symptoms, 77
AN1792, 124
antioxidants, 199, 200
APOE-e4, 182, 183
Auguste Deter, 122

brain organization, 3–11, 13–17, 19, 21, 25, 26

CAD106, 124, 125
caregiver resources, 238, 241
caregiving, 222, 223
central nervous system, 40
cerebrospinal fluid (CSF), 6, 9, 14
chronic traumatic encephalopathy (CTE), 60, 168, 169
clinical trials, 129, 131, 132, 134, 136
cognitive reserve, 52–55
concussion, 165–170
CRISPR/Cas9, 202, 203

deep-brain stimulation (DBS), 162, 163
dementia, 59–61, 63–66
diet, 229–231

differential diagnosis, 78, 79, 82
drug development, 124, 127–132, 134–136

early diagnosis, 224
early-onset Alzheimer's disease, 142–145
environment, 196
ethnicity, 100, 105
evolution, 140, 141
exercise, 194, 198, 200–202

familial Alzheimer's disease, 142, 144
frontotemporal dementia (FTD), 60

genetics, 100, 101, 111
glia, 5, 10, 12
global burden, 107

H.M., COGNIShunt, 158, 159
hormones, 100, 101

late-onset Alzheimer's disease, 143
lewy body, 81, 82
lobbying, 235, 237, 239
Low-Level Light Therapy, 203

marijuana (THC), 207
military, 169

mitosis, 43, 44
music, 211, 212, 214

National Alzheimer's Project, 111
neuroanatomy, 8
neurogenesis, 40, 41, 43, 44
neuron, 5, 10–15, 17–19
normal pressure hydrocephalus
    (NPH), 60

pathology, 32, 38
Phineas Gage, 157
Pittsburgh Compound B (PiB),
    180
plasticity, 15–17
prevalence, 99, 100, 103, 105, 107,
    110
prevention, 229
prophylactic treatment, 224, 228
protein ubiquitination, 68

risk stratification, 224, 227

90+ Study, 50
senility, 49, 51, 52
Shinya Yamanaka, 160
sleep, 146–148
smoking, 103–105
solanezumab, 135–137, 177, 178
stem cell, 159
stem cell therapy, 191
stem cell treatments, 158–161
support groups, 238, 240, 241

tau oligomer-specific monoclonal
    antibody (TOMA), 178
tau protein tangles, 89
telomere, 34
traumatic brain injury (TBI), 60, 165
trisomy 21 (Down syndrome), 145
tumor, 36, 41, 44

vascular dementia, 81
vitamin B12, 82, 83
vitamin E, 175, 176